Model-based design of optimal reactors for (bio)pharmaceutical manufacturing

MODEL-BASED DESIGN OF OPTIMAL REACTORS FOR (BIO)PHARMACEUTICAL MANUFACTURING

Von der Fakultät für Maschinenbau
der Technischen Universität Carolo-Wilhelmina zu Braunschweig

zur Erlangung der Würde

eines Doktor-Ingenieurs (Dr.-Ing.)

genehmigte Dissertation

von: M. Sc. Victor Nnamdi Emenike
aus (Geburtsort): Lagos, Nigeria

eingereicht am: 03.05.2019
mündliche Prüfung am: 04.11.2019

Gutachter:

Prof. Dr.-Ing. Ulrike Krewer
Prof. Dr.-Ing. Kai Sundmacher

2019

Bibliografische Information der Deutschen Nationalbibliothek
Die Deutsche Nationalbibliothek verzeichnet diese Publikation in der Deutschen Nationalbibliografie; detaillierte bibliographische Daten sind im Internet über http://dnb.d-nb.de abrufbar.
1. Aufl. - Göttingen: Cuvillier, 2019
Zugl.: (TU) Braunschweig, Univ., Diss., 2019

Nonnenstieg 8, 37075 Göttingen
Telefon: 0551-54724-0
Telefax: 0551-54724-21
www.cuvillier.de

1. Auflage, 2019
Gedruckt auf umweltfreundlichem, säurefreiem Papier aus nachhaltiger Forstwirtschaft.

ISBN 978-3-7369-7117-2
eISBN 978-3-7369-6117-3

To my mother, for her love, strength and unwavering support.

ACKNOWLEDGMENTS

First and foremost, I thank God almighty, the creator of heaven and earth who has helped me all through my life and in completing this thesis. God, I thank you for inspiring, guiding and giving me the strength to complete this thesis. Next, I thank my father who sadly is not here with us today. I thank you for your training, instructions, sacrifice and love. I hope the completion of this thesis makes you smile in heaven. I thank my mother who has been my rock and greatest supporter. Mum, I appreciate you for your love, support and care. Your words of encouragement, listening ears and prayers have made me the man that I am today. Thank you also mummy for standing strong for the family in the absence of daddy and for sacrificing so much so that my siblings and I can pursue our dreams.

Furthermore, I thank my supervisor Prof. Dr.-Ing. Ulrike Krewer for believing in me and giving me the opportunity to work in her lab. Ulrike, I thank you for all your advice and support that has enabled me to grow as a researcher and person. I thank you for working so hard to provide a conducive working environment for me and others at the institute, for funding my participation at conferences, and for helping me find my feet when I newly came to Germany. I still remember how you found a temporary accommodation for me and how you gave me your personal airbed. May God bless you! I thank Prof. Dr.-Ing. Kai Sundmacher for agreeing to be my second examiner and member of my PhD Advisory Committee (PAC). Your wisdom and advice during my PAC meetings are well appreciated. I also wish to thank Prof. Dr.-Ing. Andreas Seidel-Morgenstern and Dr. Ju Weon Lee for the fruitful discussion concerning their paper on the nucleophilic aromatic substitution of 2,4-difluoronitrobenzene. I appreciate Nicolas Kaiser for the helpful discussions and assistance at the onset of my PhD.

I thank all members of InES for providing a healthy work environment. Specifically, I thank the members of the PSE group. I deeply appreciate my PhD mentor, Dr.-Ing. René Schenkendorf. René, I thank you for your technical insights, words of encouragement and speedy reviews. Without your input, the quality of this thesis would be lower and the time of completion might be longer. Next, I thank other members of the PSE group, Moritz Schulze and Xiangzhong Xie. It has been awesome having you guys as team mates. I thank you for the discussions both scientific and non-scientific and for the research collaboratons. I also thank Moritz and René for assisting me in editing the German version of the abstract of this thesis. Thank you Moritz for critically reviewing the first draft of this thesis. I thank my collaborators Dominik Hertwerk, Rüdiger Ohs, and Prof. Dr.-Ing. Antje Spiess for a successful collaboration which has enriched the scope and content of this thesis. Special thanks goes to Dominik who conducted the laboratory experiments in Chapter 4 of this thesis. I gratefully acknowledge the Ministry of Science and Culture, Lower Saxony, Germany under the SynFoBiA project for providing the funding that has made most of the work in this PhD thesis possible.

I also thank Daniel Schröder who was my first office mate, for being an excellent inspiration in my first year. Thank you Fabian Kubannek for being an excellent peer-to-peer mentor especially in the early years of my PhD. I thank Ina Schunke for providing excellent administrative support and Wilfried Janßen for providing IT support. I also thank them both for being very friendly to me and for helping me practise my German.

I thank Pastor Prince Ansah and members of the Christian Hope Church Braunschweig for being a strong support group and for being a family away from home. I deeply appreciate my best friend Stephen for the gift of friendship and for being a friend that sticks closer than a brother. Thank you for always checking up on me and for pushing me to finish this PhD!

Finally, I appreciate the invaluable advice from my past teachers and mentors: Dr. Daniel Ayo and Dr. Michail Stamatakis; and the moral support from my friends: Angela, Femi, Lanre, Lesho, Momo, Nneka, Susan, Tobi, Tumi and Xorla.

Victor Nnamdi Emenike
Braunschweig
April 2019

CONTENTS

LIST OF FIGURES

LIST OF TABLES

ABSTRACT

The pharmaceutical industry is on the cusp of a technological revolution especially with regards to its manufacturing practices. At the center of this advancement, is the Quality by Design paradigm—which was initiated by the U.S. Food and Drug Administration—to guide the development of future manufacturing processes for small and large molecule drugs.

Moreover, it has been identified by academia and industry alike that process systems engineering will play a crucial role in making Quality by Design possible. A focal point of process systems engineering is a systems-oriented framework that is based on chemical engineering unit operations. While the unit operations approach has served the chemical industries, there are recent ideas for designing manufacturing processes by leveraging ideas from process intensification. A recent idea in process intensification is the concept of elementary process functions (EPF) which proposes designing processes by considering their inherent functionalities instead of already prescribed unit operations. By so doing, the optimal route in thermodynamic state space can be obtained and then technically approximated by either an appropriate off-the-shelf unit operation or could lead to the design of novel processes. So far the, EPF approach has found success specifically in the area of reactor design for the production of bulk chemicals. Therefore, the major goal of this thesis is to extend the EPF approach to design optimal reactors for pharmaceutical process development and manufacturing.

There are four main contributions in this thesis. First, it is shown how the EPF concept can be adapted to design reactors for the synthesis of active pharmaceutical ingredients—small molecule drugs—and organic intermediates. By considering the nucleophilic aromatic substitution as a case study, it is demonstrated that the residence time in comparison to results from the literature could be reduced by 33% by only exploiting the heating flux and that dosing strategies have no benefits in this case.

Second, the EPF approach was extended to enzyme-catalyzed reactions specifically benzaldehyde lyase (BAL)-catalyzed carboligation. In contrast to the preceding case study, it was shown that dosing strategies could lead to a 13% improvement of the final product concentration in comparison to a reference batch reactor. Moreover, this result was experimentally validated.

Based on this improvement, a robust optimal reactor for the BAL-catalyzed carboligation was designed as the third contribution of this thesis. In doing so, a systematic reactor design approach that combines the EPF conceptual framework, global sensitivity analysis, and a novel point estimate method-based back-off strategy was proposed. It was shown that this back-off approach could lead to the design of robust optimal reactors, while being at least 10 times faster than the conventional Monte Carlo-based back-off approach.

Lastly, the EPF approach was extended to multi-scale bioreactor design for the manufacture of biologics—large molecule drugs. As a case study, the recombinant production of erythropoietin in *Pichia pastoris* using glucose as a substrate was considered, and the dynamic flux balance analysis approach was cast into the EPF framework. Moroever, a novel solution strategy for solving such optimization problems was proposed. The approach combines ideas from simultaneous dynamic optimization, bilevel optimization and the exact ℓ_1-penalization scheme. By using this approach it was shown that both optimal extracellular and intracellular fluxes leading to a 66% improvement in productivity could be resolved efficiently in less than one second. It was shown that this improvement could be obtained by implementing an almost constant optimal feeding strategy, which is different from typical exponential feeding strategies; and the engineering of a *P. pastoris* strain with high activity of most pathways in the central carbon metabolism.

Ultimately, this thesis has shown that the EPF approach is a viable approach for designing optimal and robust reactors for the synthesis of active pharmaceutical ingredients and organic intermediates, and for manufacturing biologics.

KURZFASSUNG

Die Pharmaindustrie durchläuft einen tiefgreifenden Wandel, der durch eine technologische Revolution der Herstellungsverfahren getrieben wird. Im Mittelpunkt des Umbruches steht das Quality-by-Design, das von der amerikanischen Food and Drug Administration initiiert wurde, um die Entwicklung zukünftiger Fertigungsprozesse für nieder- und hochmolekulare Medikamente zu steuern. Basierend auf den Anforderungen der Industrie und unter Berücksichtigung der aktuellen Fachliteratur spielen systemverfahrenstechnische Konzepte (engl. Process Systems Engineering) bei der Implementierung von Quality-by-Design-Methoden eine entscheidende Rolle.

Die systemorientierte Betrachtung von verfahrenstechnischen Prozessen des „Process Systems Engineering" basiert gewöhnlich auf verfahrenstechnischen Grundoperationen (engl. Unit Operations) und deren technischen Realisierungen. Während der Unit-Operations-Ansatz in der Chemieindustrie heute bereits weit verbreitet ist, nimmt die Bedeutung von innovativen Prozessintensivierungstrategien bei der Gestaltung von Herstellungsprozessen im Bereich von Forschung und Entwicklung stetig zu. Ein vielversprechendes Prozessintensivierungskonzept ist das der Elementaren Prozessfunktionen (EPF), das als Gegenpol zum traditionellen Unit-Operations-Ansatz die verfahrenstechnische Prozessgestaltung unter Berücksichtigung von thermodynamischen Zustandsgrößen beschreibt. Auf diese Weise kann zunächst die optimale Prozess-/Syntheseroute im thermodynamischen Zustandsraum ohne technische Vorprägung und Einschränkung bestimmt werden. Erst anschließend erfolgt der Schritt der technischen Realisierung bzw. dient die berechnete optimale Syntheseroute als Grundlage für das Design von neuen verfahrenstechnischen Prozesseinheiten. Insbesondere bei der Gestaltung von Reaktoren für die Produktion von Grundchemikalien führte die erstmalig angewandte EPF-Methodik zu signifikanten Prozessverbesserungen. Basierend auf den bisher erreichten Erfolgen steht im Fokus der vorliegenden Arbeit die Erweiterung des EPF-Ansatzes auf die optimale Reaktorauslegung für die Wirkstoffherstellung.

Die erzielten Ergebnisse lassen sich in vier wesentliche wissenschaftliche Beiträge einordnen. Zunächst wird das EPF-Konzept für das Reaktordesign zur Synthese von pharmazeutischen Wirkstoffen (engl. Active Pharmaceutical Ingredients, APIs) und organischen (niedermolekularen) Zwischenprodukten angewandt. Als erste Fallstudie wird eine nukleophile aromatische Substitution betrachtet, bei der allein durch die Optimierung des Thermo-Managements die Verweilzeit um 33% reduziert werden konnte. Gleichermaßen wird gezeigt, dass eine dynamische Anregung anhand von Dosierungsstrategien keine weitere Prozessverbesserung erzielt.

Darauf aufbauend wird der EPF-Ansatz auf enzymatische Reaktionen, speziell auf Benzaldehyd-Lyase- (BAL)-katalysierte Carboligationen, ausgeweitet. Im Gegensatz zur vorangehenden Fallstudie führen hier optimierte Dosierungsstrategien zu einer Erhöhung der Produktkonzentration um 13% im Vergleich zu Versuchen im Batch-Reaktor. Eine anschließende experimentelle Validierung konnte die simulativ errechneten Ergebnisse bestätigen.

Ergänzend beinhaltet der dritte Beitrag dieser Arbeit ein robustes optimales Reaktordesign für das BAL-katalysierte Reaktionssystem. Hauptmerkmal des robusten Designkonzepts ist ein systematischer Ansatz, der die EPF-Theorie, die Analyse von globalen Sensitivitäten und eine neuartige Backoff-Strategie auf Basis der Point Estimate Method (PEM) vereint. Mit der PEM-basierten Strategie können robuste, optimale Reaktorauslegungen erzielt werden, bei denen die Rechnersimulationen zehnmal schneller konvergieren als konventionelle Monte-Carlo-basierte Ansätze.

Im letzten Beitrag wird ein Multiskalen-Ansatz erstmalig mit der EPF-Theorie verknüpft, um Herstellungsprozesse von hochmolekularen Biopharmazeutika für die Reaktorauslegung abbilden zu können. Als Fallbeispiel dient die rekombinante Produktion von Erythropoetin aus *Pichia pastoris*, bei der die dynamische Flussbilanzanalyse (dFBA) in eine EPF-basierte Optimierung eingebettet wurde. Der neue Ansatz kombiniert Lösungsstrategien aus der Bilevel- und dynamischen Optimierung mittels exaktem l_1-Penalisierungsschemas. Durch die Optimierung der inner- und außerzellularen Flussraten wird eine Produktivitätssteigerung um 66% berechnet – bei weniger als eine Sekunde Rechnerlaufzeit. Diese Verbesserung kann durch die Implementierung eines nahezu konstanten Zuflusses von Glucose-Substrat erreicht werden. Bemerkenswert dabei ist, dass das Ergebnis in starkem Kontrast zu vorherrschenden Dosierungsstrategien steht, bei denen typischerweise exponentiell dosiert wird.

Zusammenfassend zeigt diese Arbeit, dass der EPF-Ansatz ein praktikables und zielführendes Werkzeug für die Entwicklung optimaler und robuster Reaktoren zur Synthese von niedermolekularen APIs, organischen Zwischenprodukten und zur Herstellung von höhermolekularen Biopharmazeutika darstellt.

PREFACE

This work was conducted during my employment as a research associate ("Wissenschaftlicher Mitarbeiter") at the Institute of Energy and Process Systems Engineering (InES), TU Braunschweig between June 2014 and June 2018. Besides my primary affiliation with InES, I also held joint affiliations at the International Max Planck Research School for Advanced Methods in Process Systems Engineering (IMPRS ProEng) and the Center for Pharmaceutical Engineering (PVZ) at TU Braunschweig.

Moreover, the research in this thesis has been published/submitted in peer-reviewed scientific journals and presented at conferences. These journal publications and conference proceedings are listed below.

JOURNAL PUBLICATIONS

1. Emenike, V.N., Krewer, U., Model-based optimal design of continuous flow reactors for the synthesis of active pharmaceutical ingredients. Chemie Ingenieur Technik, 88(9), pp. 1215-1216, 2016.

2. Emenike, V.N., Schulze, M., Schenkendorf, R., Krewer, U., Model-based optimization of the recombinant protein production in *Pichia pastoris* based on dynamic flux balance analysis and elementary process functions. Computer Aided Chemical Engineering, 40, pp. 2815-2820, 2017.

3. Emenike, V.N., Schenkendorf, R., Krewer, U., A systematic reactor design approach for the synthesis of active pharmaceutical ingredients. European Journal of Pharmaceutics and Biopharmaceutics, 126, pp. 75 - 88, 2018.

4. Emenike, V.N., Schenkendorf, R., Krewer, U., Model-based optimization of biopharmaceutical manufacturing in *Pichia pastoris* based on dynamic flux balance analysis. Computers & Chemical Engineering, 118, pp. 1 - 13, 2018.

5. Emenike, V.N., Xie, X., Schenkendorf, R.,Spiess, A.C., Krewer, U., Robust dynamic optimization of enzyme-catalyzed carboligation: a point estimate-based back-off approach. Computers & Chemical Engineering, 121, pp. 232 - 247, 2019.

6. Emenike, V.N., Xie, X., Schenkendorf, R., Krewer, U., A point estimate method-based back-off approach to robust optimization: application to pharmaceutical processes. Computer Aided Chemical Engineering, 46, pp. 223 - 228, 2019.

7. Emenike, V.N., Hertwig, D., Schenkendorf, R., Spiess, A.C., Krewer, U., A rigorous model-driven approach for the optimal design of reaction strategies for enzyme catalysis. *In Preparation* 2019.

CONFERENCE PROCEEDINGS

1. Emenike, V.N., Krewer, U., Model-based optimal design of continuous flow reactors for the synthesis of active pharmaceutical ingredients. ProcessNet-Jahrestagung und 32. DECHEMA-Jahrestagung der Biotechnologen 2016, Aachen, Germany, 12 - 15 September, 2016.

2. Emenike, V.N., Schulze, M., Schenkendorf, R., Krewer, U., Model-based optimal design of reactors for biopharmaceutical manufacturing of recombinant proteins in *Pichia pastoris*. 15th International Conference on Molecular Systems Biology (ICMSB2017), Raitenhaslach, Munich, Germany, 26 - 28 July, 2017.

3. Emenike, V.N., Schenkendorf, R., Krewer, U., Advances in model-assisted process design for (bio)pharmaceutical manufacturing. 2nd International Symposium on Pharmaceutical Engineering Research (SPhERe), Braunschweig, Germany, 6 - 8 September, 2017.

4. Emenike, V.N., Schulze, M., Schenkendorf, R., Krewer, U., Model-based optimization of the recombinant protein production in *Pichia pastoris* based on dynamic flux balance analysis and elementary process functions. 10th World Congress of Chemical Engineering (WCCE10)/ 27th European Symposium on Computer Aided Process Engineering (ESCAPE-27), Barcelona, Spain, 1 - 5 October, 2017.

5. Emenike, V.N., Hertwig, D., Schenkendorf, R., Krewer, U., Spiess, A. Out-of-the-box process intensification for enzyme-catalyzed cross-carboligation. 12th Symposium of the European Society of Biochemical Engineering Sciences (ESBES2018), Lisbon, Portugal, 9 - 12 September, 2018.

6. Emenike, V.N., Xie, X., Schenkendorf, R., Krewer, U., A point estimate method-based back-off approach to robust optimization: application to pharmaceutical processes. 29th European Symposium on Computer Aided Process Engineering (ESCAPE-29), Eindhoven, Netherlands, 16 - 19 June, 2019.

1

INTRODUCTION

The pharmaceutical industry has for centuries served as a vanguard for producing high quality medicines for the well-being of humanity. Traditionally, the quality of these medicines have been ensured by using procedural guidelines [37]. These guidelines have been set-up by regulatory bodies such as the United State's Food and Drug Administration (FDA) and the European Medicines Agency. The major driver for these guidelines as set by both institutions stems from historical issues regarding the toxicity of drugs and manufacturing failures in the 1960s and 1970s [37]. A classical example is an incident in 1932, where diethylene glycol which is toxic to humans, was used to produce the elixir of sulfanilamide [77]. Another classical example was the sulfathiazole disaster in 1941 which was found to be due to poor manufacturing practises as documented in [179].

Due to these issues, the FDA established a forerunner of the current Good Manufacturing Practices (cGMPs) in the early 1960s and later finalized it in 1978. From then on, pharmaceutical companies have endeavoured to meet these cGMPs by following procedural regulatory control measures which are based on quality by testing [37, 144].

Due to economic constraints, it has been agreed by industry leaders and regulatory bodies alike that areas of pharmaceutical manufacturing ranging from clinical trials to actual drug production have to be modernized. Due to this, the International Conference on Harmonization introduced the process analytical technology (PAT) and Quality by Design (QbD) initiatives about 15 years ago [37]. QbD entails using PAT tools such as sensors to ensure and monitor critical quality attributes and quality target product profiles by manipulating critical process parameters [98].

Even though QbD is relatively new to the pharmaceutical industry, the inherent technologies in QbD have already been widely applied in the chemical and petrochemical industries. As such, there is a rising campaign for the pharmaceutical manufacturers to adopt QbD. Nevertheless, a successful implementation of QbD involves the implementation of technologies such as PAT [167], continuous manufacturing [37] and process systems engineering [59].

Moreover, it is envisioned that process systems engineering—a subdomain of chemical engineering—will play a pivotal role in designing future pharmaceutical processes [182, 59]. A key goal of this thesis is to cross-fertilize the domains of process systems engineering and pharmaceutical manufacturing.

Based on this short background on the history of pharmaceutical manufacturing, the motivation for the specific research conducted in this thesis will be presented in the subsequent sections. By doing so, the aim is to give the reader a background knowledge in pharmaceutical manufacturing and the role of chemical engineering in pharmaceutical manufacturing. Ultimately, the research hypothesis, objectives and structure of the thesis will be presented in the final sections of this chapter.

1.1 PHARMACEUTICAL MANUFACTURING

Traditionally,[1] batch processing is the standard in the fine chemicals and pharmaceutical industry because of its simplicity and flexibility [150]. However, batch manufacturing has some well-known disadvantages such as scale-up difficulties, mass and heat transfer bottlenecks, long production times and possible supply chain disruptions [153, 149]. As shown in Fig. 1.1, the multiple disconnected steps involved in batch pharmaceutical manufacturing are the major causes of the long production times and possible supply chain disruptions.

[1] This section has been published in Emenike *et al.*, Eur. J. Pharm. Biopharm. 2018, 126, 75-88 [50].

Continuous pharmaceutical manufacturing (CPM) , in turn, is a process intensification strategy that enables the reduction of the number of synthesis steps and units, which can lead to significant cost savings [158, 85]. Furthermore, CPM enables safer operation [149, 63, 60], better scalability, enhanced process automation, smaller process footprint, enhanced mass and heat transfer, and higher throughput [98]. As a result, CPM is considered by both academia and industry as the most viable alternative to batch manufacturing [81]. To demonstrate the merits of CPM, Mascia *et al.* [110] developed an end-to-end continuous pharmaceutical manufacturing plant that produces drug products in final tablet form from chemical intermediates. The illustration of this end-to-end CPM plant can be seen in Fig. 1.2.

At the heart of the shift from batch to CPM technology are continuous flow reactors (or simply flow reactors), which serve as the key driver of highly-intensified flow processes; and they can be intensified by using elevated temperatures and pressures, light or immobilization agents [197, 10]. Hence, flow reactors are currently being used to synthesize APIs [20, 61] and organic intermediates quite frequently [170]. Based on the advantages of flow reactors, Hessel proposed the concept of novel process windows, i.e. operating under extreme process conditions to improve API production [68].

However, Valera *et al.* [184] argued that the advantages cited for flow reactors might not always be the case and that the decision to operate a reaction continuously or batch-wise should be done on a case-by-case basis. Hence, the question arises: *how do we systematically choose the best reactor type for a particular API synthesis?*

In an attempt to answer this question, Plouffe *et al.* [136] proposed a tool box approach for the selection of the best reactor for a particular reaction based on reaction classes, reacting phase (single or multiphase), and the reaction network. However, the authors admitted that this heuristic-based approach might not encompass all reaction types [136]. Model-based approaches such as attainable region methods [72] and superstructure-reactor optimization [1] could be used, but these methods are still dependent on existing reactor types, i.e. following a component off-the-shelf philosophy.

Inspired by this challenge, this thesis proposes the use of an apparatus-independent methodology called elementary process functions (EPF) developed by Freund and Sundmacher [56, 132]. A model-based approach such as the EPF methodology can guide the optimal design of intensified flow reactors and complement synthesis experiments. This can lead to novel process windows [68]; thereby, accelerating the pharmaceutical process development phase.

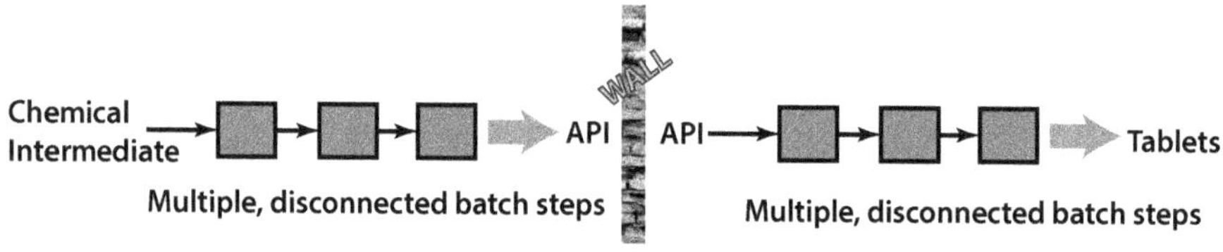

Figure 1.1: Batch pharmaceutical manufacturing.

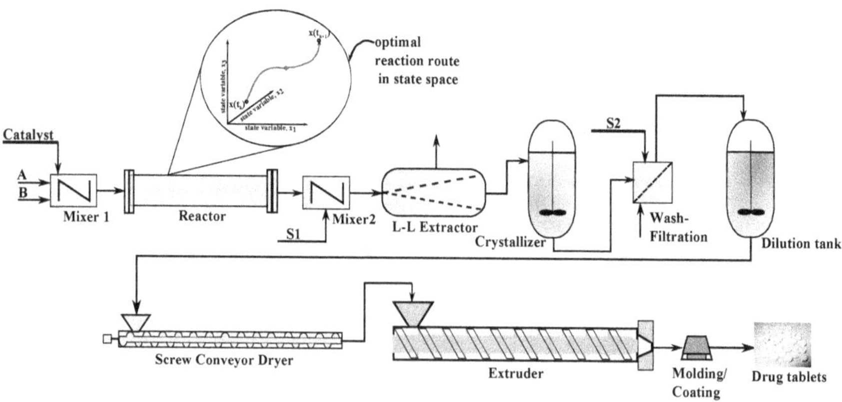

Figure 1.2: Continuous pharmaceutical manufacturing.

1.2 CHEMICAL REACTION ENGINEERING FOR API SYNTHESIS

In recent times,[2] chemical reaction engineering (CRE) concepts are increasingly being applied to design reactors for the synthesis of active pharmaceutical ingredients (APIs) and organic intermediates [120, 198, 84]. For example, Shukla *et al.* [166] applied CRE principles to maximize the selectivity of a diazotization reaction in continuous flow reactors. Jolliffe and Gerogiorgis applied CRE and other process engineering tools to design a conceptual process for the continuous manufacturing of ibuprofen [84] and artemisinin [86]. By applying CRE tools, Nagy *et al.* [120] derived simple heuristics for determining when it is important to consider dispersion or mixing in flow reactor design, dimensioning, and scale-up. Witt *et al.* [198] compared models of varying complexity for the design of mesoscale flow reactors. Westermann and Mleczko [196] applied CRE principles to highlight the importance of considering heat management (which is usually ignored) in the design of continuous flow reactors for organic synthesis. However, the aforementioned studies are based on the selection of "off-the-shelf" reactors; thus, limiting the possibility of novel reactors or the selection of the best existing reactor.

Moreover, chemical engineers and chemists in pharmaceutical drug development rely on established types of flow reactor during their modelling and simulation or laboratory protocols. As described by Roberge [136, 151], there are three basic flow reactors used in API synthesis, namely: plug flow (coil) reactors, continuous-stirred tank reactors (CSTRs) , and plate reactors. Furthermore, new types of reactors such as the multi-injector reactor [8, 152], the continuous oscillatory baffled reactor [177], the agitated cell reactor [27], and the filter reactor [36] have been developed and applied to CPM. Experimentally, it is almost impossible to compare all possible candidates of flow reactors for a particular synthesis protocol due to cost and time constraints. Even for a small subset of available reactors at the lab scale, it is infeasible to consider all possible reactor configurations in the design space

---

[2]This section has been published in Emenike *et al.* 2018 [50].

and to determine the underlying optimal operating conditions by means of experimental trial-and-error.

Furthermore, most of the continuous flow reactor modelling activities reported in the current literature are based on simulations with little or no model-based optimization studies. Even though a number of optimization-based reactor design approaches exist [1, 72], these methods still depend on established reactor types. Therefore, the possibilities for the optimal design of new intensified reactors are limited. Here, an apparatus-independent concept such as the elementary process functions (EPF) might be an interesting alternative. In this work, the focus is on demonstrating how the EPF approach can be used to design optimal reactor configurations for API synthesis problems.

1.3 RESEARCH HYPOTHESIS AND OBJECTIVES

The research hypothesis of this thesis can be posited as follows:

"The elementary process functions methodology can be used to design optimal reactors for the synthesis of active pharmaceutical ingredients and biopharmaceuticals."

The objectives of this thesis are as follows:

1. To develop reactor design methods based on the EPF philosophy for (bio)pharmaceutical manufacturing.
2. To develop tailored process systems engineering methods that are based on EPF for (bio)pharmaceutical manufacturing.

Therefore, the aim of this thesis to cross-fertilize knowledge in the domains of systematic methods for reactor design, pharmaceutical manufacturing and PSE.

1.4 THESIS STRUCTURE

The structure of this thesis starts off with Chapter 2 where the main methodologies used in this thesis are discussed. The following four chapters (Chapter 3 - 6) present the main contributions of this thesis. Chapter 7 concludes the thesis. The subsequent chapters are summarized as follows.

Chapter 2 - Methodology. The EPF methodology is discussed in detail and the simultaneous approach that is used to solve all resulting dynamic optimization problems in this thesis is also described.

Chapter 3 - A systematic reactor design approach for the synthesis of active pharmaceutical ingredients. This provides a demonstration of how the EPF methodology can be applied to design reactors for API synthesis. As a case study, an organic synthesis reaction was considered; namely, the nucleophilic aromatic substitution of 2,4-difluoronitrobenzene. At the end of this chapter, it is intended that the reader will have gotten a thorough overview of how the EPF approach can be adapted to design reactors for the synthesis of APIs.

Chapter 4 - Model-based design of an optimal reactor for enzyme catalyzed cross-carboligation. This chapter further extends the applicability of the EPF methodology to the field of biocatalysis and apply it specifically to enzyme-catalyzed carboligation. In contrast to Chapter 3 which is purely computational; here, an experimental validation is provided that demonstrates that the EPF approach can indeed lead to novel designs that improve the pharmaceutical manufacturing process.

Chapter 5 - Robust dynamic optimization of enzyme-catalyzed carboligation. Following up on the reactor designs from Chapter 4; which were obtained under the assumption that the parameters are certain, the reactor design problem in the presence of parametric uncertainty is considered.

Chapter 6 - Multiscale bioreactor design based on dynamic flux balance analysis. Prior to this chapter, the focus has been on reactor design at the mesoscale level (i.e. the reactor level) and also on the synthesis of small molecule drugs or organic intermediates. Here, the manufacturing of biologics; large molecule drugs, is considered. Furthermore, the reactor design problem will be integrated and addressed on two scales; namely, the microorganism and bioreactor scales.

Chapter 7 - Conclusions and future directions. This chapter provides a general summary of the whole thesis, and presents open research questions and possible ideas that could be pursued in the future.

2

METHODOLOGY

In this chapter,[3] the two key methods used throughout this thesis are presented and described in some detail. These two methods are the elementary process functions and dynamic optimization. First, the elementary process functions approach to designing processes, particularly reactors, will be delineated. The mathematical formulation of the elementary process functions approach typically results in an a dynamic optimization problem.

Therefore, the approach used in solving the dynamic optimization problems that appear throughout this thesis will be described in detail. There are various methods for solving dynamic optimization problems but only the simultaneous approach is used in this thesis. As such, the reason why the simultaneous approach was used instead of other competing methods will be presented.

2.1 ELEMENTARY PROCESS FUNCTIONS

The elementary process functions (EPF) framework proposed by Freund and Sundmacher [56] is a main workhorse of this thesis. The EPF approach differentiates itself from the conven-

[3]Parts of this chapter have been published in Emenike *et al.*, Eur. J. Pharm. Biopharm. 2018, 126, 75-88 [50] and Emenike *et al.*, Comput. Chem. Eng. 2019, 121, pp. 232 - 247 [52].

tional unit-operation approach which is usually based on "off-the-shelf" processing units such as mixers, reactors, distillation columns, etc. The key idea is to replace such processing units with functional modules and track a fluid element travelling through these functional modules. In each functional module, e.g. a reaction module, the changes of the state (e.g. mass, energy, concentration, etc.) of a fluid element with time are influenced by fluxes (controls) such as heat fluxes, component dosing fluxes, diffusion fluxes, etc (see Fig. 2.1). Mathematically, the fluid element is represented as [56]:

$$\frac{\mathrm{d}\mathbf{x}}{\mathrm{d}t} = \sum_{k=1}^{J} j_k^{\Phi}(\mathbf{x}) \cdot \mathbf{e}_k, \tag{2.1}$$

where $\mathbf{x}$ is a state vector, j_k^{Φ} is the flux k of the functional module Φ, $\mathbf{e}_k$ is the EPF of flux k, i.e., its basis vector in thermodynamic state space, and J is the total number of fluxes of the functional module Φ. The EPF $\mathbf{e}_k$ represents a certain direction of the flux k in thermodynamic state space, and the combined effect of the EPFs determines the region in thermodynamic state space that is attainable by the fluid element (see [56] for details). Alternatively, Eq. (2.1) could be re-written in state-space representation notation as:

$$\frac{\mathrm{d}\mathbf{x}}{\mathrm{d}t} = \mathbf{E}(\mathbf{x}) \cdot \mathbf{j}^{\Phi}(\mathbf{x}), \tag{2.2}$$

where $\mathbf{j}^{\Phi}$ is the generalized flux vector of the functional module Φ, and $\mathbf{E}$ is the elementary process functions matrix which is the product of the inverse capacity matrix and a flux weighting matrix (see [131] for details).

Based on the EPF approach, Peschel *et al.* [132] developed a systematic reactor design methodology. Here, the optimal reaction route in state space with respect to a particular objective function is obtained. Examples of these objective functions include minimal residence time, highest possible conversion or selectivity. As a result, various process intensification methods can be incorporated into the reactor design process. In literature, it has been shown that this concept can lead to novel intensified optimal reactors [132, 133, 134].

In the sequel, the three levels of the EPF-based reactor design approach—integration and enhancement, control variable selection, and technical approximation—will be described. For a more detailed discussion, the reader is referred to [132] and references therein.

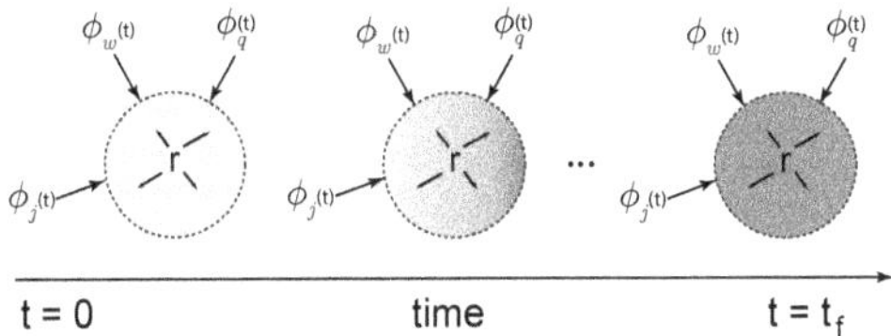

Figure 2.1: Conceptual representation of a fluid element in thermodynamic state space affected by generic time-varying component dosing fluxes $\phi_j(t)$ and $\phi_w(t)$, the reaction flux r, and heat flux $\phi_q(t)$.

Level 1: Integration and enhancement

On the first level, process intensification concepts [175] such as integration and enhancement are considered. Here, integration refers to a unit with more than one function e.g. reactive distillation column; while enhancement involves the use of fluxes such as heat flux and component dosing fluxes to improve the process. Typically, the intensification concepts are chosen based on the reactor designer's experience, but a more systematic approach such as the superstructure optimization concept [1] might be implemented as well at this stage. Furthermore, the optimal reaction route is obtained under the influence of fluxes optimized along the path of the fluid element, and no limitations arising from predefined reactors are imposed. The only constraints are due to thermodynamic relations, reaction kinetic, and system-inherent features such as temperature bounds and solubility.

The dynamic behaviour of the representative fluid element is modelled by the Lagrangian approach [7] to incorporate the non-geometric and apparatus-independent nature of EPF. Moreover, this formulation leads to short computation times and relatively fast screening of various process intensification (PI) options with the purpose of identifying an optimal reaction route [132]. Ultimately, the goal of the first level is to determine the best theoretically possible reaction route which will serve as a benchmark for the next two levels and any final reactor implementation.

Level 2: Control variable selection

At the second level, technically implementable control variables are selected to approximate the pre-defined flux profiles from level 1. This is because heat flux and component dosing fluxes can be limited by heat transfer kinetics and mass transfer kinetics in reality.

Furthermore, the flow regime, a particular channel geometry, and a prototype reactor set-up is assumed at this level. Finally, the best control variables that lead to an optimal objective value close to that of the first level are selected, and realized in the third level.

Level 3: Technical approximation

The technical approximation can be achieved by using off-the-shelf reactors or by novel design principles based on the optimal reaction route and related control profiles from the previous levels. Nevertheless, it should be mentioned that the technical approximation of the reaction route and control profiles are not unique but are dependent on the engineering judgement of the reactor designer.

It is also possible to consider different hypothetical technical reactors within a superstructure framework [1] comparing various configurations simultaneously. As soon as a suitable reactor design is chosen, simple and rigorous reactor models can be formulated and optimized in order to ascertain the optimal fine-tuned configuration of the identified reactor. Lastly, the three levels led to a class of mathematical problems called dynamic optimization problems. The details of the solution approach used to solve them can be found in 3.3.

2.2 DYNAMIC OPTIMIZATION: MATHEMATICAL FORMULATION

The design problem within the EPF framework translates into a dynamic optimization problem where fluxes flowing in and out of the fluid element are optimized as the fluid element is tracked in thermodynamic state space. In this thesis, the focus will be on a Mayer-type problem [18] with the following general form:

$$
\begin{aligned}
\underset{\mathbf{x}(\cdot),\mathbf{u}(\cdot),\mathbf{z}(\cdot)}{\text{minimize}} \quad & \Phi(\mathbf{x}(t_\mathrm{f})) \\
\text{subject to} \quad & \dot{\mathbf{x}}(t) = \mathbf{f}(\mathbf{x}(t),\mathbf{z}(t),\mathbf{u}(t),\boldsymbol{\theta}), \quad \forall t \in \mathcal{T}, \\
& \mathbf{g}(\mathbf{x}(t),\mathbf{z}(t),\mathbf{u}(t),\boldsymbol{\theta}) = \mathbf{0}, \quad \forall t \in \mathcal{T}, \\
& \mathbf{h}(\mathbf{x}(t),\mathbf{z}(t),\mathbf{u}(t),\boldsymbol{\theta}) \leq \mathbf{0}, \quad \forall t \in \mathcal{T}, \\
& \mathbf{x}(t_0) = \mathbf{x}_0, \\
& \mathbf{u}(t) \in \mathcal{U},
\end{aligned}
\tag{2.3}
$$

on the time horizon $\mathcal{T} := [t_0, t_\mathrm{f}] \subset \mathbb{R}$, where t_0 and t_f are the initial and final time points, respectively. The control vector $\mathbf{u} \in \mathbb{R}^{n_u}$ is an element of the admissible set of controls $\mathcal{U}$; $\Phi(\mathbf{x}(t_\mathrm{f}))$ is an objective function which is to be minimized (or maximized); $\mathbf{x}(t) \in \mathbb{R}^{n_\mathrm{x}}$ is a vector of state variables; $\mathbf{z}(t) \in \mathbb{R}^{n_\mathrm{z}}$ is a vector of algebraic variables; $\boldsymbol{\theta} \in \mathbb{R}^{n_\theta}$ is a vector of time-independent parameters; $\mathbf{f} : \mathcal{T} \times \mathbb{R}^{n_\mathrm{x}} \times \mathbb{R}^{n_u} \times \mathbb{R}^{n_\mathrm{z}} \times \mathbb{R}^{n_\theta} \rightarrow \mathbb{R}^{n_\mathrm{x}}$ is a function vector that defines the derivatives of the states; $\mathbf{g} : \mathcal{T} \times \mathbb{R}^{n_\mathrm{x}} \times \mathbb{R}^{n_u} \times \mathbb{R}^{n_\mathrm{z}} \times \mathbb{R}^{n_\theta} \rightarrow \mathbb{R}^{n_\mathrm{g}}$ is a function vector that defines the equality constraints; $\mathbf{h} : \mathcal{T} \times \mathbb{R}^{n_\mathrm{x}} \times \mathbb{R}^{n_u} \times \mathbb{R}^{n_\mathrm{z}} \times \mathbb{R}^{n_\theta} \rightarrow \mathbb{R}^{n_\mathrm{h}}$ is the inequality (path) constraint function vector; and $\mathbf{x}_0$ is a vector of the initial conditions of the states at initial time t_0 which could also be decision variables.

2.3 DYNAMIC OPTIMIZATION SOLUTION STRATEGY

There are three main approaches for solving the dynamic optimization problem defined in Eq. (2.3), namely: dynamic programming, indirect, and direct approaches [155]. Dynamic programming [12] typical is not suitable for large scale problems because it suffers from the "curse of dimensionality" [102, 155]. Indirect ("optimize-then-discretize") methods such as Pontryagin's minimum principle [138] are also known to be unapplicable to large scale problems because of difficulties in handling adjoints associated with path constraints [155]. Direct ("discretize-then-optimize") methods are usually the method of choice for complex, highly nonlinear, large scale problems [155] such as the those considered in this thesis. Direct methods include single shooting (a.k.a. control vector parameterization) [185, 186], multiple shooting [19], and the simultaneous approach (a.k.a. direct collocation) [16].

To solve the infinite dimensional dynamic optimization problem (2.3), the simultaneous approach is employed to discretize the states and control of the problem (2.3) to get a finite-dimensional nonlinear programming (NLP) problem [15, 40]. The simultaneous approach was selected because it allows us to transcribe Eq. (2.3) directly into NLPs without the need for successively calling a DAE solver as is the case for both control vector parameterization and multiple shooting [17]. Furthermore, the simultaneous approach has been shown to handle instabilities and path constraints efficiently [17, 18]. In particular, a direct collocation method is used; where the time horizon is discretized into finite elements N with each element containing K collocation points. The method is depicted pictorially on Fig. 2.2. Here, the states $\mathbf{x}$ and algebraic variables $\mathbf{z}$ are discretized on the finite elements and the collocation points by parameterizing them with orthogonal polynomials on Radau collocation points, while the controls $\mathbf{u}$ are discretized on only the finite elements by using a piecewise constant parameterization. First, an ordered set of indices is defined for the finite elements as $\mathcal{F} = \{1, \dots, N\}$ and that of the collocation points as $\mathcal{C} = \{1, \dots, K\}$ and then present the discretized form of problem (2.3) as the following NLP problem:

$$\underset{\hat{\mathbf{x}},\hat{\mathbf{u}},\hat{\mathbf{z}}}{\text{minimize}} \quad \Phi(\mathbf{x}_N) \tag{2.4a}$$

$$\text{subject to} \quad \dot{\mathbf{x}}_{i,j} = \mathbf{f}(\mathbf{x}_{i,j}, \mathbf{z}_{i,j}, \mathbf{u}_i, \boldsymbol{\theta}), \quad \forall i \in \mathcal{F}, j \in \mathcal{C}, \tag{2.4b}$$

$$\mathbf{x}_{i,j} = \mathbf{x}_i + \sum_{k=1}^{K} \boldsymbol{\Omega}_{k,j} \dot{\mathbf{x}}_{i,j}, \quad \forall i \in \mathcal{F}, j \in \mathcal{C}, \tag{2.4c}$$

$$\mathbf{g}(\mathbf{x}_{i,j}, \mathbf{z}_{i,j}, \mathbf{u}_i, \boldsymbol{\theta}) = \mathbf{0}, \quad \forall i \in \mathcal{F}, j \in \mathcal{C}, \tag{2.4d}$$

$$\mathbf{h}(\mathbf{x}_{i,j}, \mathbf{z}_{i,j}, \mathbf{u}_i, \boldsymbol{\theta}) \leq \mathbf{0}, \quad \forall i \in \mathcal{F}, j \in \mathcal{C}, \tag{2.4e}$$

$$\mathbf{x}_1 = \mathbf{x}_0, \tag{2.4f}$$

$$\mathbf{x}_{i+1} = \mathbf{x}_{i,K}, \quad \forall i \in \mathcal{F} \backslash \{N\}. \tag{2.4g}$$

For the sake of a compact representation of the decision variables, the discretized states, algebraic variables, and controls are collected into separate vectors:

$$\hat{\mathbf{x}} := \begin{bmatrix} \mathbf{x}_1 \\ \mathbf{x}_{1,1} \\ \vdots \\ \mathbf{x}_{N,K-1} \\ \mathbf{x}_N \end{bmatrix}, \qquad \hat{\mathbf{z}} := \begin{bmatrix} \mathbf{z}_{1,1} \\ \vdots \\ \mathbf{z}_{N,K-1} \\ \mathbf{z}_{N,K} \end{bmatrix}, \qquad \hat{\mathbf{u}} := \begin{bmatrix} \mathbf{u}_1 \\ \vdots \\ \mathbf{u}_N \end{bmatrix},$$

with $\mathbf{x}_i, \mathbf{x}_{i,j} \in \mathbb{R}^{n_x}$, $\mathbf{z}_{i,j} \in \mathbb{R}^{n_z}$, and $\mathbf{u}_i \in \mathbb{R}^{n_u}$. The discretized form of the Mayer-type objective function (2.4a) is now defined at the last finite element N and collocation point K as $\Phi(\mathbf{x}_N)$, and Eq. (2.4b) represents the discretized differential states. Furthermore, the collocation equations over the finite elements $i \in \mathcal{F}$ and collocation points $j \in \mathcal{C}$ are defined by Eq. (2.4c). These equations utilize parameters from the collocation matrix $\boldsymbol{\Omega}$ which is derived from an orthogonal polynomial of order K with roots at Radau collocation points [18]. Eqs. (2.4d) and (2.4e) define the equality constraints and path constraints over $i \in \mathcal{F}$ and $j \in \mathcal{C}$, respectively. Finally, Eq. (2.4f) defines the initial point, while Eq. (2.4g) enforces the continuity of the differential profiles.

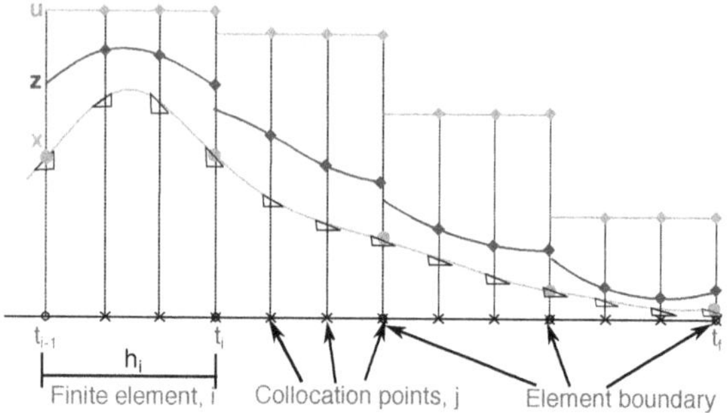

Figure 2.2: The simultaneous approach: direct collocation on finite elements (adapted from [17]). The diamonds represent the controls **u** and algebraic variables **z** at the collocation points. The triangles represent the slope of the states $\dot{\mathbf{x}}$ on the collocation points, and the circles represent the states **x** at the boundaries of the finite element. **u** is represented by a piecewise constant discretization on the finite elements, while **x** and **u** are parameterized by orthogonal polynomials on both the finite elements and collocation points. Furthermore, discontinuities are allowed for **u** and **z**, while continuity is enforced for **x**.

3

A SYSTEMATIC REACTOR DESIGN APPROACH FOR THE SYNTHESIS OF ACTIVE PHARMACEUTICAL INGREDIENTS

The focus of this chapter is to demonstrate the adaptation of the three-level reactor design methodology described in Chapter 2 to the synthesis of active pharmaceutical ingredients and organic intermediates. This chapter is a modified version of the published work [50].

This chapter is organized as follows: in Section 3.1, the reaction mechanism and reaction kinetics of the case study, the nucleophilic aromatic substitution of 2,4-difluoronitrobenzene is presented. In Section 3.2, the model formulation and results for the first level of the reactor design procedure are presented. In Section 3.4, the model formulation and results for the second level of the reactor design procedure are presented. In Section 3.5 a technical reactor is proposed based on the results from Section 3.2 and 3.4. Computational details on the dynamic optimization are presented in Section 3.3 and the chapter is finally summarized in Section 3.6.

3.1 OPTIMAL REACTOR DESIGN FOR THE NUCLEOPHILIC AROMATIC SUBSTITUTION OF 2,4-DIFLUORONITROBENZENE

As a case study of pharmaceutical relevance, a homogeneous liquid phase nucleophilic aromatic substitution (S_NAr) of 2,4-difluoronitrobenzene in the presence of morpholine

[100] is considered. The EPF approach is applied to design an optimal reactor design for the S_NAr reaction of 2,4-difluoronitrobenzene. This model reaction was chosen because of its pervasive utility in the pharmaceutical industry [123, 145, 34] and the availability of kinetic data [100].

The related reaction kinetics and mechanism used in this work was adapted from the work by Lee *et al.* [100] (see Fig. 3.1). The reaction scheme for this reaction is shown in Fig. 3.2 where 2,4-difluoronitrobenzene **1** reacts with morpholine **2** to produce the target ortho product **3**, a para by-product **4**, by-product **5**, and a charged molecule **6**.

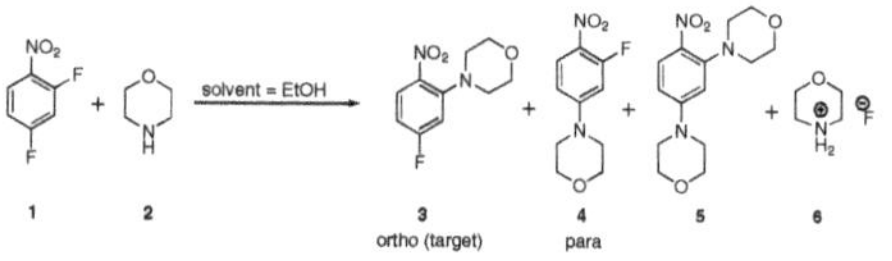

Figure 3.1: Reaction scheme for the nucleophilic aromatic substitution of 2,4-difluoronitrobenzene (**1**) with morpholine (**2**) to produce the ortho regio-selective isomer **3**, para regio-selective isomer **4** and by-products **5** and **6**.

According to reference [100], it was assumed that species in charged ionic form are negligible. O'Brien and co-workers also reported that the salt byproduct **6** was removed by an extraction process [123]. Hence, **6** would not be considered in the reaction mechanism as shown in Fig. 3.2. Furthermore, hydrogen fluoride (HF) is assumed not to be in the gaseous form as it can form ionic bonds with the amine groups of the reaction products and reactant **2** [100]. HF can also form alcohol–HF mixtures with the ethanol solvent as stated in Reference [112]. However, these were not considered in this study in order to keep the model complexity tractable. These assumptions are also supported with the fact that the reactions were handled in the homogeneous liquid phase by Lee *et al.* [100]. The objective of this work is to design an optimal reactor that minimizes the residence time of the S_NAr reaction between 2,4-difluoronitrobenzene (**1**) and morpholine (**2**). The corresponding decision structure for the reactor design procedure is shown in Fig. 3.3 and explained in more detail in the sequel.

$$1 + 2 \xrightarrow{k_1} 3 + HF$$

$$1 + 2 \xrightarrow{k_2} 4 + HF$$

$$3 + 2 \xrightarrow{k_3} 5 + HF$$

$$4 + 2 \xrightarrow{k_4} 5 + HF$$

Figure 3.2: Reaction mechanism for the nucleophilic aromatic substitution of 2,4-difluoronitrobenzene.

3.2 LEVEL 1: APPLYING INTEGRATION AND ENHANCEMENT CONCEPTS

In this chapter, three intensification cases (see Fig. 3.3) were considered with the objective to minimize the residence time of the studied reaction system. These include:

1. Reactor intensification by heat-flux/reaction temperature optimization as a generic concept for minimizing the residence time [54].

2. For the remaining two cases, the concept of component flux dosing is considered. This intensification method was chosen because dosing strategies may lead to reduced residence times while leading to better temperature control and mitigation of hot spots [152, 64].

For the sake of comparison, the proposed options are benchmarked against an optimal reference case from literature [100]. Here, an isothermal tubular (coiled) flow reactor was optimized by simulation and experimental studies. The optimal residence time, temperature, feed-ratio of morpholine (**2**)-to-2,4-difluoronitrobenzene (**1**), and selectivity was 5 minutes, 393.15 K, 2.7, and 87 %, respectively. Next, each intensification and enhancement concept considered is explained in more detail.

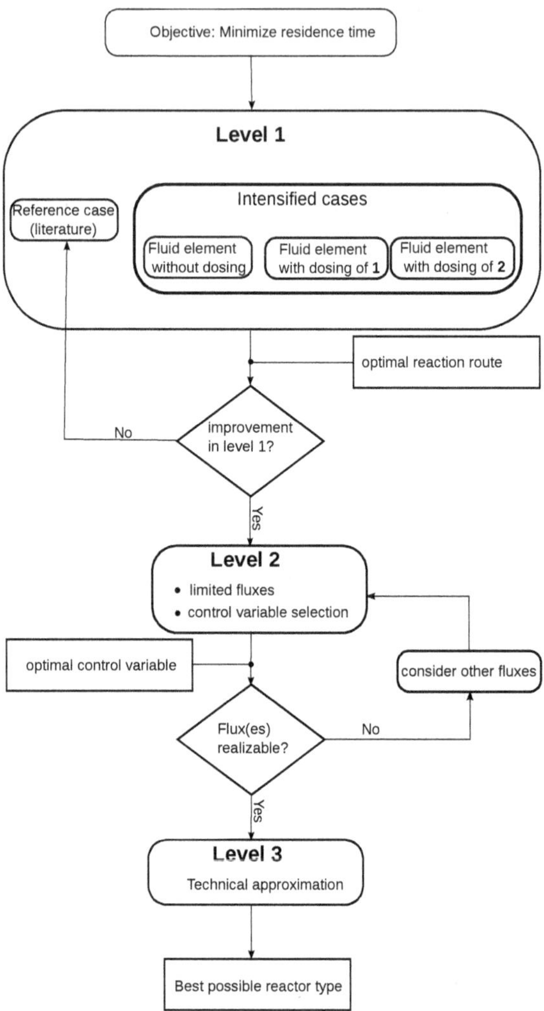

Figure 3.3: EPF decision structure for the intensified reactor design.

Case 1: Fluid element without dosing

In this case, the feed ratio and heat flux are optimized assuming ideal unconstrained fluxes (on the first level). Technically, heat flux changes are mimicked by using the reactor temperature as the control variable while the feed ratio will be considered as an additional design parameter.

Case 2: Fluid element with dosing of **1**

Case 2 is similar to case 1, with the addition of another control variable: the component dosing flux of reactant **1** along the reaction route. This enables us to consider the possibility of an enhancement concept that involves the interplay between the optimal heat flux and reactant **1** dosing profiles.

Case 3: Fluid element with dosing of **2**

Case 3 follows the same idea as case 2, but with reactant **2** dosed along the reaction coordinate instead of reactant **1**. This strategy enables us to consider the effect that the optimal heat flux and reactant **2** dosing will have on the residence time.

Model development for the EPF level 1

The mole balances are formulated by using the Lagrangian approach. Furthermore, the reaction was assumed to be carried out entirely in the liquid phase and the solvent volume was assumed to be equal to or larger than the volume of reacting species. Thus, the densities of each component and the volume of the fluid element were assumed to be constant. The concentration for the solvent, ethanol is considered as a constant, while the mole balances for the other reaction components i (see Fig. 3.1) are given as:

$$\frac{dn_i(t)}{dt} = \mathbf{s}^{c^\top} \cdot \mathbf{j}(t) + \sum_{m}^{N_{\text{reac}}} \nu_{i,m} \cdot r_m \cdot V \quad \forall i \in \{\mathbf{1}, \mathbf{2}\}, \tag{3.1}$$

$$\frac{dn_i(t)}{dt} = \sum_{j}^{N_{\text{reac}}} \nu_{i,m} \cdot r_m \cdot V \quad \forall i \in \{\mathbf{3}, \mathbf{4}, \mathbf{5}, \text{HF}\}, \tag{3.2}$$

where $\mathbf{j}(t) := [j_1(t), j_2(t)]^\top$ is a vector representing the component dosing fluxes with $j_1(t)$ and $j_2(t)$ representing dosing of **1** and **2**, respectively. $\mathbf{s}^c$ is a selection vector which determines the dosing fluxes are considered in each case $c \in \{1, 2, 3\}$. $\mathbf{s}^c$ is set as $[0, 0]$, $[1, 0]$ and $[0, 1]$ for cases 1, 2, and 3, respectively. $\nu_{i,m}$ is a stoichiometric ratio of component i in reaction m, r_m is the rate of reaction m and V is the volume of the fluid element. Typically, the volume is formulated as a function of the number of moles, temperature dependent density, and molecular weight of the reaction species [67]. However, with the unavailability of temperature dependent density equations for the $S_N Ar$ reaction molecules, a constant volume of 10 mL [100] has been assumed in this study. This assumption is plausible since significant volume changes in small scale systems with a single organic phase is not expected. Furthermore, the stoichiometric ratios $\nu_{i,m}$ follow the reactions in Fig. 3.2. The reaction rates r_m are expressed by power law kinetics as postulated by Lee *et al.* [100] according to:

$$r_m = k_m \prod_{i}^{N_{\text{comp}}} C_i^{||\nu_{i,m}||} \quad \forall m \in N_{\text{reac}} \tag{3.3}$$

where N_{comp} is the number of reacting components, N_{reac} is the number of reactions and the rate constants k_m for each reaction m is given by the Arrhenius equation:

$$k_m = k_{\infty,m} exp\left(\frac{-E_{\text{A},m}}{RT}\right) \tag{3.4}$$

where $k_{\infty,m}$ and $E_{\text{A},m}$ are the pre-exponential factor and activation energy for reaction m, respectively. The values for $k_{\infty,m}$ and $E_{\text{A},m}$ were taken from [100] and are given in Table 3.1.

Lastly, performance measures such as conversion $\mathcal{X}$ and selectivity $\mathcal{S}$ are presented below:

$$\mathcal{X} = \frac{n_{1,\text{tot}} - n_{1,0}}{n_{1,\text{tot}}} \tag{3.5}$$

$$\mathcal{S} = \frac{n_{3,f} - n_{3,0}}{\mathcal{X} \cdot n_{1,\text{tot}}} \tag{3.6}$$

where $n_{1,tot}$ is the sum of the initial amount and dosed amount of 2,4-difluoronitrobenzene, and $n_{3,f}$ is the final amount of the target product at the end of the reaction.

Table 3.1: Reaction kinetic parameters taken from Lee *et al.* [100].

Reaction	k_∞ [L/(mol min)]	E_A [J/mol]
r_1	1.8673×10^6	43.6×10^3
r_2	1.7514×10^4	35.8×10^3
r_3	9.7012×10^3	40.4×10^3
r_4	6.1063×10^8	70.1×10^3

Optimization formulations for level 1

A case-dependent dynamic optimization formulation for minimizing the residence time τ is described as:

$$\underset{T(t),\, \mathbf{s}^\top \mathbf{j}(t),\, n_{1,0},\, \gamma}{\text{minimize}} \quad \tau \tag{3.7a}$$

$$\text{subject to} \quad \text{Mole balances : Eqs. (3.1) and (3.2),} \tag{3.7b}$$

$$\text{Reaction rates : Eqs. (3.3) and (3.4),} \tag{3.7c}$$

$$\text{Performance measures : Eqs. (3.5) and (3.6),} \tag{3.7d}$$

$$\text{Terminal constraints} : \mathcal{X} = 0.99, \tag{3.7e}$$

$$\text{Intrinsic bounds} : \; T \in [T_\text{L}, T_\text{U}],\; \gamma \in [\gamma_\text{L}, \gamma_\text{U}], \tag{3.7f}$$

$$\text{System bounds} : \; \mathcal{S} \in [0,1],\; n_{i,\text{tot}} = n_{i,0} + \int_0^\tau j_i dt \;\; \forall i \in \{\mathbf{1},\mathbf{2}\}, \tag{3.7g}$$

$$\text{Case specific selection vector} : \; \mathbf{s}^\text{c}. \tag{3.7h}$$

In addition to the residence time, other objective functions such as the yield maximization [132], selectivity maximization [134], space time yield maximization [46] or even multi-objective functions can be evaluated depending on the problem at hand. In this work, the conversion was set at 99 % to avoid challenges in downstream separation [100]. As conversion is nearly complete ($\mathcal{X} = 0.99$) and is set as a terminal constraint, it is not expedient to use the final conversion as an objective function. Furthermore, preliminary studies using the selectivity as the objective function were conducted and it was found that the selectivity and yield cannot be improved as explained in the next section. Therefore, the residence time was selected as the objective function for this study.

The temperature range, 353.15 to 393.15 K at which the kinetic experiments were performed were used to define the lower bound T_L and upper bound T_U on the temperature control variable. Similarly, the upper and lower bounds of the feed-ratio γ of reactant 2 to 1 were chosen as $\gamma_L = 1$ and $\gamma_U = 3$, respectively. This was done in order to ensure that the reaction kinetics remain valid through out the optimization procedure. Please note, to ensure a fair comparison with the literature reference case, these constraints are applied here as well.

3.3 IMPLEMENTATION

The dynamic optimization problems formulated at level 1 and the subsequent levels were transcribed into large scale NLP problems by using the simultaneous dynamic optimization solution approach described in Section 2.3.

50 finite elements and three collocation points were used to transcribe the dynamic optimization problems to NLPs. The resulting NLPs were implemented in the algebraic mathematical language AMPL [55] by using the CONOPT solver [44]. All computations were performed on a PC running a CentOS operating system with an Intel(R) Core(TM) i7-4789 processor at 3.60 GHz, and 16 GB RAM.

Results for level 1

The dynamic optimization result of the first case in level 1 is shown in Fig. 3.4. The concentration profiles and temperature control profile are shown in Fig. 3.4a and 3.4b, respectively. The residence time for the first case (i.e. no dosing) in level 1 is 3.22 minutes which is a 35 % decrease from the reference case [100] that was optimized by combining experiments and simulations. It can be seen in Fig. 3.4b that the temperature profile remains at the upper bound of 393.15 K. This is due to the fact that the reaction would ideally be completed in the shortest possible time if it operates at the highest possible temperature throughout the course of the reaction. The temperature profiles of the second and third cases (i.e. dosing of **1** and **2**) are equal to that of the first case and thus not shown here. Nevertheless, the temperature profile implies that operating at the maximum temperature leads to the shortest residence time. Also, the ratio of reactant **2** to reactant **1** for the case 1 is 3 to 1, i.e. the upper bound.

The intensification strategies at level 1 show that the dosing of reactants does not lead to lower residence times or higher selectivity (see A.1 and Fig. A.1 and A.2). This is due to the fact that the reaction order of reactants **1** and **2** are the same in the desired and undesired reactions. Hence, the dependence of reaction rates on the concentration of reactants **1** and **2** in the desired and undesired reactions are the same.

Moreover, the reactions are all irreversible and purely driven by the kinetics and not by thermodynamics. This kind of reaction is termed neutral as reported in Lu *et al.* [107] and Hamel *et al.* [65]. Therefore, the only way to minimize the residence time is to exploit the heat flux and feed ratio of reactants **1** and **2**.

In the next section, the aim is to implement the idealized heat flux obtained by incorporating an energy balance that includes transport kinetics to obtain realistic heat fluxes.

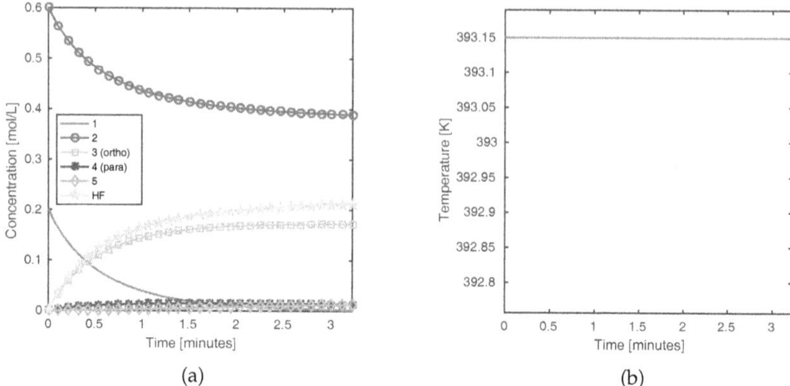

Figure 3.4: Optimization results for the first level in the case of the fluid element without dosing (τ = 3.22 minutes, γ = 3.00): a) concentration state profiles; b) temperature control profile.

3.4 LEVEL 2: LIMITED FLUXES AND CONTROL VARIABLE SELECTION

In level 2, the major goal is to select physically implementable control variables that can approximate the control profiles obtained in level 1. That is, transport kinetic limitations on the heat flux in terms of material and environmental factors are added.

Model development for level 2

In addition to the model equations in level 1, an energy balance is included as shown below:

$$\left(\frac{\sum_i^{N_{\text{comp}}} n_i c_{\text{p},i}}{V_{\text{reac}}} + \frac{\rho_{\text{EtOH}} \cdot c_{\text{p,EtOH}}}{\text{Mwt}_{\text{EtOH}}}\right)\frac{dT}{dt} = -\left(a \cdot j_{\text{q}} + \sum_m^{N_{\text{reac}}} r_m \cdot \Delta H_m\right) \tag{3.8}$$

where $c_{\text{p},i}$ is the temperature-dependent specific heat capacity of component i in J/(mol K) which is derived from group contribution methods [147]—please see Section A.3 of Appendix A for more details. V_{reac} is the total volume of the reacting species (excluding the solvent) in L, and ρ_{EtOH} is the density of the solvent (ethanol) in g/L. Mwt_{EtOH} is the molecular weight of ethanol in g/mol, a $(= 4/d_{\text{t}})$ is the surface-to-volume ratio in mm^2/mm^3, and j_q is the heat flux in $J/(s\,m^2)$. The standard enthalpies of reactions ΔH_m were taken from Reference [100]. The heat flux j_q transport kinetics is assumed to follow Fourier's law and it is given as:

$$j_q = h(T - T_e) \tag{3.9}$$

where h is the heat transfer coefficient which is kept constant at 0.5 $kW/(m^2\,K)$ as done in [134], and T_e is the environment (heating or cooling) temperature in Kelvin (K). For details on the model development of the energy balance for level 2, the reader is referred to Appendix A.2.

Optimization formulations for EPF level 2

The optimization formulation of level 2 has the same structure as that of level 1, but with changes in the state and control vectors, and with additional variables and constraints. Since an energy balance is on the second level, the reaction temperature is now considered as a state variable and not as a control variable.

Moreover, the volume of the solvent V_{EtOH} is chosen as a decision variable within reasonable bounds and the volume of the reacting species V_{reac} is constrained by the equality constraint:

$$V_{reac} = V - V_{EtOH} \tag{3.10}$$

Furthermore, a soft constraint was included to minimize the heat loss by limiting the difference between the initial temperature T_0 and final temperature T_f to a maximum of 1 K as done in [169] and [104]:

$$(T_f - T_0)^2 \leq 1 \tag{3.11}$$

Due to the small volume of the reactor considered in this work, the corresponding bound on the tube diameter was set between 1 to 1.5 mm [197, 94]. Therefore, the optimization of the second level is given as follows:

$$\underset{T_e(t), d_t, V_{EtOH}, n_{1,0}, \gamma}{\text{minimize}} \quad \tau \tag{3.12a}$$

$$\text{subject to} \quad \text{Mole balances : Eqs. (3.1) and (3.2),} \tag{3.12b}$$

$$\text{Energy balance : Eq. (3.8),} \tag{3.12c}$$

$$\text{Heat flux transport kinetics : Eq. (3.9),} \tag{3.12d}$$

$$\text{Reaction rates : Eqs. (3.3) and (3.4),} \tag{3.12e}$$

$$\text{Performance measures : Eqs. (3.5) and (3.6),} \tag{3.12f}$$

$$\text{Volume constraint : Eq. (3.10),} \tag{3.12g}$$

$$\text{Terminal constraint :} \mathcal{X} = 0.99, \tag{3.12h}$$

$$\text{Heat loss constraint : Eq. (3.11),} \tag{3.12i}$$

$$\text{Intrinsic bounds : } T \in [T_L, T_U],\ T_e \in [T_{eL}, T_{eU}],\ \gamma \in [\gamma_L, \gamma_U], \tag{3.12j}$$

$$\text{Design bounds : } d_t \in [d_{tL}, d_{tU}], \tag{3.12k}$$

$$\text{System bounds : } \mathcal{S} \in [0, 1] \tag{3.12l}$$

The bounds of the reaction temperature are similar to those of level 1, while the environment temperature T_e is set to reasonable bounds from 300 to 393.15 K. The parameters and bounds used in the optimization formulation for level 2 are summarized in Table 3.2.

Results for level 2

In the case of limited kinetics, the minimum residence time and selectivity for the reaction are approximately 3.31 minutes and 87 %, respectively. This slight increase in residence time of about 2.9 % is due to Eq. 3.11 and the non-idealities incorporated in level 2. Obviously, the environment temperature is a suitable control variable for implementing the reaction route and corresponding control profiles. Furthermore, the optimal solvent volume, tube diameter and the feed ratio obtained are 5 mL, 1 mm and 3.0, respectively.

Table 3.2: Optimization parameter values used in level 2 .

Parameters	values	units
h	0.5	$\mathrm{kW/(m^2\,K)}$
T_0	353.15	K
T_{L}	353.15	K
T_{U}	393.15	K
T_{eL}	353.15	K
T_{eU}	393.15	K
γ_{L}	1	-
γ_{U}	3	-
d_{tL}	1	mm
d_{tU}	1.5	mm

The concentration profiles are nearly identical to those of case 1 in level 1 (cf. Fig. 3.4) while the heat flux and temperature profiles are shown in Fig. 3.5 and 3.6, respectively. The temperature profile rises from the initial temperature of 353.15 K to the upper bound, 393.15 K within the first 15 seconds and remains at the upper bound for approximately 3 minutes until the 99 % conversion condition is fulfilled. Subsequently, the temperature decreases to 354.15 K in the shortest possible time in order to fulfill the heat loss constraint (Eq. 3.11). The heat flux profile shows the initial heating of the reaction fluid to its maximum allowable temperature, followed by a zero heat flux due to no temperature gradient between the reaction temperature and environment temperature, and then cooling in the last step. This temperature profile was caused by the environment temperature which remains at its highest value of 393.15 K for the first 3.21 minutes before switching to its lower bound of 353.15 K (cf. Fig. 3.7).

As seen, the temperature has a strong impact on the residence time. Therefore, to quantify additional factors a sensitivity study was applied as shown below.

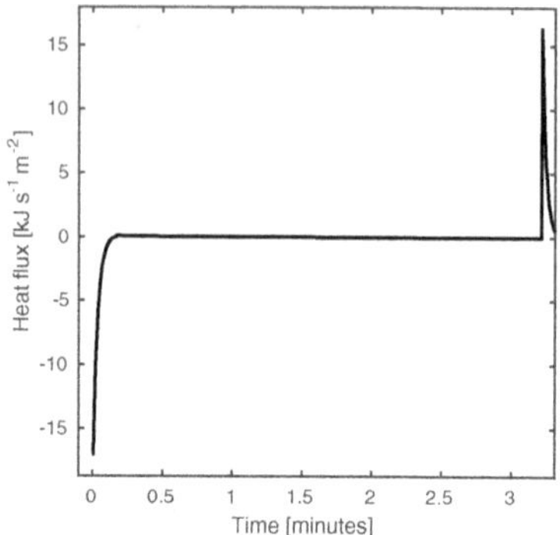

Figure 3.5: Heat flux profile for EPF level 2.

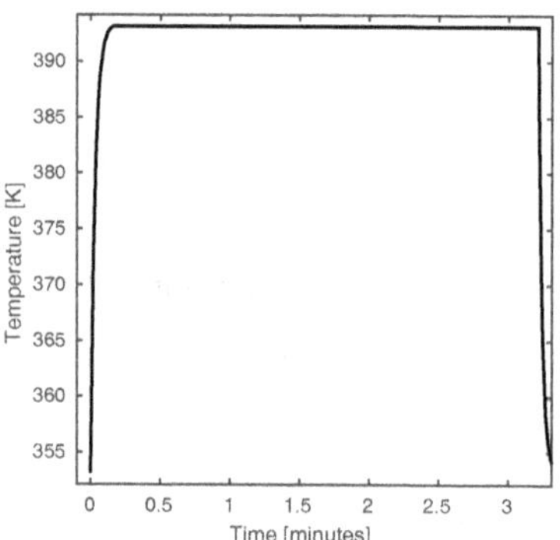

Figure 3.6: Temperature state profile for EPF level 2.

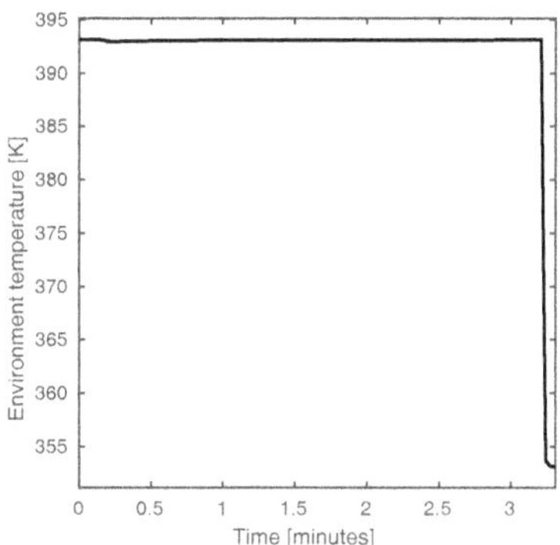

Figure 3.7: Environment temperature control profile for EPF level 2.

Parameter sensitivity analysis

In this section, a parameter sensitivity analysis on the selected case in level 2 is performed in order to determine the effect of certain design parameters before moving on to the technical approximation. The heat transfer coefficient and tube diameter were selected as two parameters of interest– as these would determine the material and the cost of the resulting technical reactor, respectively. Another important reason for a sensitivity study is to ensure that the aforementioned parameter ranges and assumed values in level 2 do not affect the model and objective adversely.

Firstly, the sensitivity analysis was performed by varying the heat transfer coefficient, h between 0.5 to $5\,\mathrm{kW}/(\mathrm{m}^2\,\mathrm{K})$ as reported by Kockmann *et al.* [94], while the diameter was kept at the constant optimal value of 1.0 mm. For a selected value of h within this interval (see Fig. 3.8a), an optimization problem was solved to determine the corresponding residence time and selectivity. Fig. 3.8a shows that increasing the heat transfer coefficient reduces the residence time, and that the selectivity remains at a constant value of approximately 86.4 % over the whole range. Moreover, the residence time between 3 to $5\,\mathrm{kW}/(\mathrm{m}^2\,\mathrm{K})$ remains at a constant value of 3.25 minutes and does not reach the 3.22 minutes attained in level 1. This is because of the additional constraint Eq. 3.11 and the fixed initial temperature of 353.15 K on level 2. Another reason is that the reaction temperature is a state variable and not a control variable in level 2.

In addition, a parameter sensitivity analysis was performed by varying the internal tube diameter, d_t between 0.1 to 2 mm [94, 100], while the heat transfer coefficient was kept at the constant previously assumed value of $0.5\,\mathrm{kW/(m^2\,K)}$. Similar to the sensitivity analysis for the heat transfer coefficient, optimization problems were solved at selected values of d_t within this interval and the corresponding residence time and selectivity for each scenario are shown in Fig. 3.8b. Obviously, the tube diameter does not have a significant impact on the selectivity. However, the residence time increases linearly with increasing tube diameter.

Based on the sensitivity analysis, it suffices to say that the selected constant heat transfer coefficient ($h = 0.5\,\mathrm{kW/(m^2\,K)}$) will be sufficient for the technical approximation in level 3; while, the tube diameter will be kept as a decision variable because it influences the residence time.

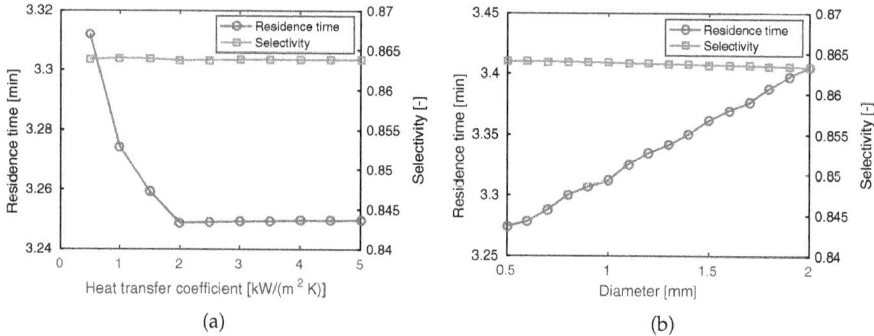

Figure 3.8: Sensitivity analysis for the environment temperature control case in EPF level 2: a) effect of heat transfer coefficient on residence time and selectivity; b) effect of tube diameter on residence time and selectivity.

3.5 LEVEL 3: TECHNICAL APPROXIMATION

In this section, an optimal technical reactor that approximates the control profiles derived in level 2 is designed. In the previous level, the environment temperature control was selected as the best control variable for the optimal reaction route of the S_NAr reaction. Based on Fig. 3.5, 3.6 and 3.7, the heat flux of the best technical reactor can be approximated by first heating, maintaining the reaction temperature at the upper bound, and then cooling for the last 2.4 seconds. However, the time required for heating and cooling are relatively small when compared to the period of constant temperature. Hence, the technical reactor is further simplified by first using a pre-heater to heat the reactants to the maximum possible temperature; feeding the reactants into a tubular reactor that is maintained at the maximum temperature by a controller, and then using the controller to switch to cooling as soon as 99 % conversion is achieved. Therefore, only the tubular reactor section will be modelled in detail and optimized in the following sections.

Furthermore, it is assumed that the best technical reactor for this reaction has plug flow characteristics as a majority of small scale reactors are assumed to have these characteristics. To identify the optimal configuration of the technical reactor, the governing equations are derived in the next step.

Model development for EPF level 3

Assuming no axial mixing, a constant reactor volume of 10 mL and an average fluid velocity, the continuous tubular coil reactor can be modelled as a one-dimensional plug-flow reactor with a heat exchanger. First, the component mole balances are given as:

$$\frac{dn_i}{dz} = \frac{V}{v} \sum_{m}^{\mathrm{N_{reac}}} \nu_{i,m} \cdot r_m \quad \forall i \in N_{\mathrm{comp}}, \tag{3.13}$$

where v is the mean fluid velocity. Furthermore, the energy balance for the reacting fluid inside the tubular reactor is given as:

$$v \cdot \left(\frac{\sum_i^{N_{\text{comp}}} n_i c_{\text{p},i}}{V_{\text{reac}}} + \frac{\rho_{\text{EtOH}} \cdot c_{\text{p,EtOH}}}{\text{Mwt}_{\text{EtOH}}} \right) \frac{dT}{dz} = -\left(a \cdot j_{\text{q}} + \sum_m^{N_{\text{reac}}} r_m \cdot \Delta H_m \right) \tag{3.14}$$

In contrast to level 2, the environment temperature (cooling/heating temperature) is not considered as a control variable. Rather, a balance is done over the environment temperature T_{e} as shown below:

$$\frac{dT_{\text{e}}}{dz} = K_{\text{e}} \cdot j_{\text{q}} \tag{3.15}$$

where K_{e} is an aggregated cooling/heating fluid-dependent parameter that ranges from -1 to $1\,\text{m K/W}$ (see Appendix A.4 and References [132] and [133]).

Furthermore, the reaction fluid velocity and flow regime is constrained by the Reynolds number:

$$\text{Re} = \frac{\rho_{\text{EtOH}} \cdot v \cdot d_{\text{t}}}{\mu_{\text{EtOH}}} \tag{3.16}$$

Other dimensionless numbers such as the Damköhler, Fourier, or Bodenstein number might be considered leading to more informed choices of the reactor types as suggested by Nagy *et al.* [120]. More details on the model formulation in level 3 can be found in A.4.

Optimization formulations for EPF Level 3

Besides the DAE model developed in Section 3.5, the volume constraint (Eq. 3.10), reasonable bounds on the Reynolds number Re, the parameter K_{e} and the mean fluid velocity v are also included in the optimization for level 3. The heat transfer coefficient was kept at a constant value of 0.5 kW/(m^2 K).

Based on the above specifications, the optimization formulation for level 3 is given as:

$$\underset{l, v, d_{\text{t}}, V_{\text{EtOH}}, n_{1,0}, \gamma}{\text{minimize}} \quad \tau \tag{3.17a}$$

$$\text{subject to} \quad \text{Mole balances : Eq. (3.13),} \tag{3.17b}$$

$$\text{Energy balance : Eq. (3.14),} \tag{3.17c}$$

$$\text{Coolant energy balance : Eq. (3.15),} \tag{3.17d}$$

$$\text{Reaction rates : Eqs. (3.3) and (3.4),} \tag{3.17e}$$

$$\text{Performance measures : Eqs. (3.5) and (3.6),} \tag{3.17f}$$

$$\text{Volume constraint : Eq. (3.10),} \tag{3.17g}$$

$$\text{Reactor length : } l = 4 \cdot V/(\pi d_{\mathrm{t}}^2), \tag{3.17h}$$

$$\text{Terminal constraint :} \mathcal{X} = 0.99, \tag{3.17i}$$

$$\text{Heat loss constraint : } (T_f - T_0)^2 \leq 1, \tag{3.17j}$$

$$\text{Intrinsic bounds : } T \in [T_{\mathrm{L}}, T_{\mathrm{U}}],\ T_{\mathrm{e}} \in [T_{\mathrm{eL}}, T_{\mathrm{eU}}],\ \gamma \in [\gamma_{\mathrm{L}}, \gamma_{\mathrm{U}}], \tag{3.17k}$$

$$\text{Design bounds : } d_{\mathrm{t}} \in [d_{\mathrm{tL}}, d_{\mathrm{tU}}], \mathrm{Re} \in [\mathrm{Re}_{\mathrm{L}}, \mathrm{Re}_{\mathrm{U}}], \tag{3.17l}$$

$$\text{System bounds : } \mathcal{S} \in [0, 1]. \tag{3.17m}$$

The optimization parameters and variable bounds used in level 3 are the same as those of level 2, with the exception of the lower and upper bound of the Reynolds number which were set at $\mathrm{Re}_{\mathrm{L}} = 100$ and $\mathrm{Re}_{\mathrm{U}} = 7000$, respectively. These bounds were chosen to keep the flow between the laminar and transition regimes. Note that the reactor length l is left as a free variable.

Results for level 3

The minimum residence time, selectivity, and optimal design variables for level 3 are summarized in Table 3.3. These results imply that the small-scale coil tubular reactor proposed in level 3 is able to technically approximate the optimal reaction route obtained in previous levels quite well. The residence time at level 3 is slightly longer than that of level 2 because of the introduction of more non-idealities. In order to determine possible materials that could be used to fabricate the reactor, a rough *back-of-the-envelope* calculation can be performed ($k \simeq h \times d_{\mathrm{t}} \sim 0.70\ \mathrm{W/(m\,K)}$). Thus, a stainless steel material can be used for the optimal technical reactor [58]. Furthermore, $K_e = 0$ as shown on Table 3.3 implies cooling at a constant temperature [131].

Moreover, the concentration profiles in level 3 are similar to those on level 2 and as such are not shown. The heat flux profile shows rapid heating from -15.88 to $0.099\,\mathrm{kJ/(s\,m^2)}$ until position 0.58 m in order to fulfill 99 % conversion (see Fig. 3.9). Following this, the heat flux decreases gradually to 0.003 $\mathrm{kJ/(s\,m^2)}$ at position 5.90 m since the reaction now generates sufficient heat to sustain itself. At 5.90 m, 99 % conversion is attained and then the heat flux switches to cooling mode.

As a result, the reaction and environment temperatures decrease after position 5.90 m as shown in Fig. 3.10 and 3.11, respectively. This behaviour is to ensure that the reaction still maintains the 99 % conversion while minimizing the energy costs. Furthermore, cooling at the tail-end of the reactor could be important if a subsequent reactor or separation unit operates at a temperature lower than the maximum temperature (393.15 K) of the S_NAr reaction.

Table 3.3: Optimal objective and design variables results for level 3.

Variable name	values	units
Residence time , τ (objective)	3.36	minutes
Selectivity, S	86	%
Feed ratio , γ	3:1	-
Heating fluid constant, K_e	0	m K/W
Internal tube diameter, d_t	1.42	mm
Reactor length, l	6.3	m
Fluid velocity, v	31.14	mm/s
Reynolds number, Re	7000	-

3.6 SUMMARY

In summary, it has been demonstrated that the elementary process functions (EPF) approach can be used to design optimal reactors for the synthesis of API and organic intermediates. As a model reaction, the S_NAr reaction of 2,4-difluoronitrobenzene with mor-

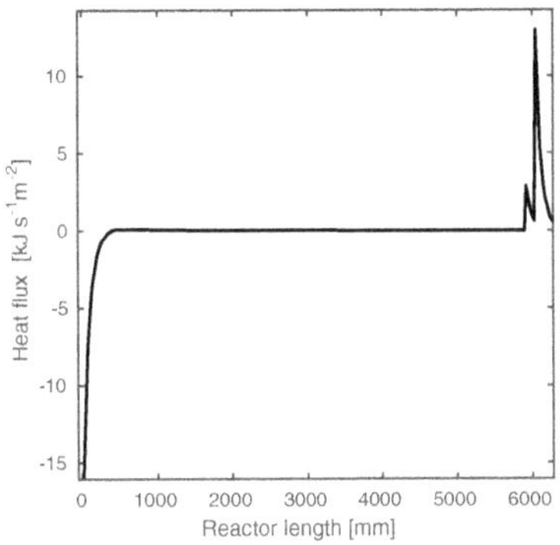

Figure 3.9: Heat flux profile for the EPF level 3.

pholine was considered; and it was shown that the EPF approach leads to optimal design outcomes in terms of a specified objective function.

The applicability of the EPF concept for any given process of interest is often hampered by the scarcity of available experimental data. To adapt the EPF approach to a particular API synthesis, the minimum required data are: a detailed reaction mechanism network, temperature-dependent reaction kinetic data, and the operating window in which the experiments were conducted.

In addition, information such as thermodynamic equilibrium data, physico-chemical properties of the reacting mixtures, fluid transport properties and a good engineering judgement will greatly improve the reliability of the results obtained by the EPF approach. Therefore, it is concluded that the successful implementation of such an approach will require close collaboration and dialogue between process systems engineers and process chemists. Indeed, as the typical data provided by chemists or pharmaceutical researchers is insufficient for the EPF approach, additional reaction engineering experiments are required.

Nevertheless, unlike other simulation-based approaches and heuristics currently used in designing reactors for API synthesis, the approach presented herein inherits the apparatus-independent nature of the EPF concept. Even though the approach led to an existing reactor

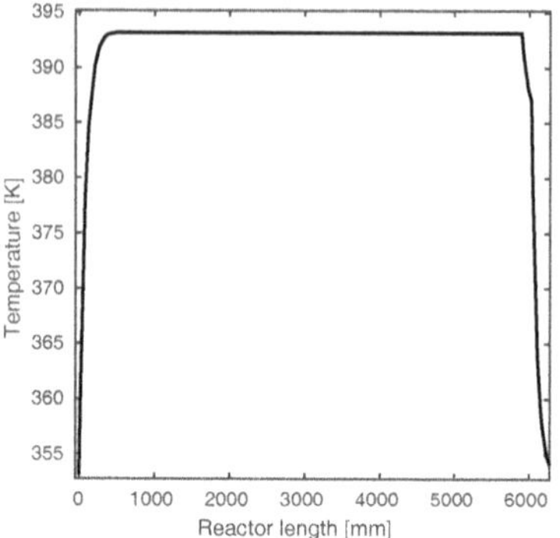

Figure 3.10: Temperature state profile for the EPF level 3.

design in this case, it also has the advantage of leading to novel reactor designs [133, 134].

In conclusion, applying the EPF approach for the design of reactors for API synthesis can lead to novel process windows [68]. Therefore, the approach can complement the experiments performed by process or organic chemists and speed-up the drug development process significantly.

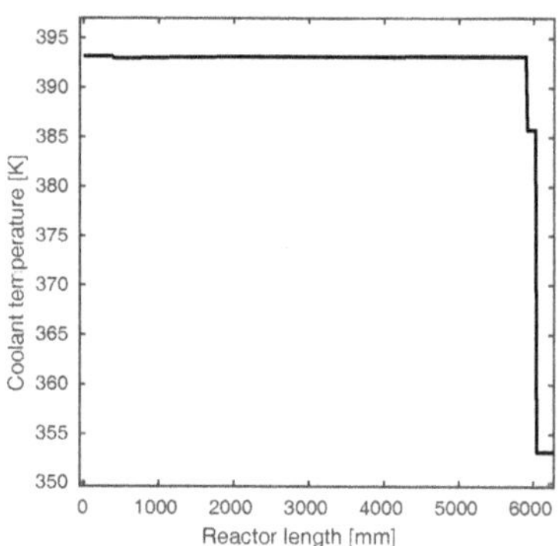

Figure 3.11: Environment temperature control profile for the EPF level 3.

4

MODEL-BASED DESIGN OF AN OPTIMAL REACTOR FOR ENZYME CATALYZED CROSS-CARBOLIGATION

This chapter further extends the applicability of the EPF methodology to the field of biocatalysis. Specifically, the EPF approach is applied to enzyme-catalyzed carboligation for the production of the pharmaceutically relevant 2-hydroxy ketones. Modified contents of this chapter can be found in [51]. In contrast to Chapter 3 which is purely computational, here, an experimental validation is presented that demonstrates that the EPF can indeed lead to novel designs that improve the pharmaceutical manufacturing process. In contrast to Chapter 3, this chapter shows that dosing intensification concepts can lead to optimal reactor designs with improved productivity metrics.

This chapter is organized as follows: in Section 4.1, a brief background pertaining to enzyme-catalyzed reactions and their reactors thereof is presented. The reaction mechanism, intensification cases, model formulation are presented in Section 4.2. The results are presented and discussed in Section 4.3, and the chapter is concluded in Section 4.4.

4.1 BACKGROUND

The pharmaceutical industry is considering biocatalytic processes as a possible alternative to chemocatalytic processes [99, 137, 199]. This is majorly due to the high stereoselectivity and specificity associated with biocatalytic processes; thus, making it possible to easily and efficiently produce high quality APIs in fewer synthesis steps [137, 199]. Fewer synthesis steps, in turn, are of economic importance to the pharmaceutical industry as less complex synthesis could translate to cost savings and greener pharmaceutical processes [199]. In the last few years, the design of biocatalysts for the efficient synthesis of APIs has witnessed tremendous advancements [99]. These advancements can be attributed to progress in protein engineering where fit-for-purpose enzymes have been designed for never-before-seen APIs [5, 99] by leveraging advanced computational methods for protein structural modeling [92], high throughout screening [35] and efficient algorithms for processing experimental data [154].

A very important class of biocatalytic reactions are C-C bond forming carboligation reactions catalyzed by thiamine diphosphate (ThDP)-dependent enzymes such as benzaldehyde lyase (BAL), benzoylformate decarboxylase (BFD) , pyruvate decarboxylase (PDC) and phenylpyruvate decarboxylase (PhPDC) [118]. These reactions usually involve reactions between aliphatic and/or aromatic aldehydes in the presence of ThDP-dependent enzymes to form optically pure 2-hydroxy ketones. 2-Hydroxy ketones are of great utility in drug production because they serve as key organic intermediates for preparing a vast array of APIs [71, 176]. Amongst the ThDP dependent enzymes, benzaldehyde lyase from *Pseudomonas fluorescens* (*Pf*BAL) is of particular interest due to its ability to conduct both carboligation and cleavage of hydro ketones [206]. However, for *Pf*BAL-catalyzed processes to be economically viable, high product concentration and low enzyme cost should be ensured [137]. As a result, these processes have to be optimized by combining knowledge from the domains of protein engineering [99], reaction engineering [148], process intensification and process engineering [91, 200]. An established way of performing this optimization is by carrying out numerous laborious experiments which are cost and time-intensive.

Therefore, computer-aided model-based approaches have been proposed to complement laboratory experiments; thus enabling cost and time savings [24, 160]. Examples of the application of model-based approaches to optimize enzyme-catalyzed reactions have already been documented in the literature. For instance, Stillger *et al.* [176] used a model-based approach to simulate and design an enzyme-membrane continuous stirred tank reactor (CSTR) for the carboligation of benzaldehyde and acetaldehyde catalyzed by *Pf*BAL to produce (*R*)-2-hydroxy-1-phenylpropanone (HPP). Parallel to this work, Hildebrand *et al.* [71] investigated the production of HPP by *Pf*BAL in a membrane CSTR using a kinetic model to simulate different reaction engineering strategies. In their work enzyme inactivation was observed and attributed to a possible reaction between the aliphatic aldehyde and the amino acids of the *Pf*BAL protein. Unfortunately, enzyme inactivation was not included in their kinetic model and thus, could not be predicted or simulated [71].

Begemann *et al.* [11] used a model-based approach to analyze reactors and develop a control strategy for a two-phase biocatalytic oxidoreduction system. Based on simulations of their model, they showed that a fed-batch reactor performed better than a batch reactor for the chosen reaction. Their simulations also showed that controlling the pH could increase conversions and improve productivity. By performing simulations with coupled kinetic models and reactor design equations, Braun *et al.* [24] minimized the enzyme costs for the biocatalytic production of 12-ketochenodeoxycholic acid in a batch reactor. Marpani *et al.* [109] utilized a kinetic model and simulation approach to determine the optimal operating conditions for the biocatalytic conversion of formaldehyde to methanol in a batch reactor. Even though their work showed excellent agreement between the simulation and experimental results, it involved performing hundreds of simulations [109]. This approach is time-consuming and could lead to sub-optimal results [50]. Furthermore, there are no rational guarantees that the design space explored by the simulations leads to optimal results.

In this chapter, the EPF approach is shown to be a viable and rigorous method for designing an optimal reactor for enzyme-catalyzed carboligation. First, various intensification strategies are investigated by using the first level of the EPF-based reactor design methodology proposed by [132]. As a case study, the *Pf*BAL-catalyzed carboligation of propanal and benzaldehyde to form (*R*)-2-hydroxy-1-phenylbutan-1-one was selected. Here, the objective is to maximize the final concentration of (*R*)-2-hydroxy-1-phenylbutan-1-one while optimally tuning the fluxes due to substrate feeding and reaction rates. This reaction was chosen because of the complex interaction between the substrate-dependent increase in reaction rates and simultaneous decrease of *Pf*BAL activity. In contrast to existing model-based studies for enzyme-catalyzed carboligation [176, 71], a detailed kinetic model that considers enzyme inactivation [125] was used. Moreover, the model-based EPF approach and laboratory experiments were successfully combined to design and validate an optimal reactor for enzyme-catalyzed carboligation.

4.2 METHODOLOGY

Reaction mechanism

The reaction mechanism for the *Pf*BAL-catalyzed conversion of propanal and benzaldehyde can be described as three coupled reaction pathways (see Fig. 4.1). In an initial step, benzaldehyde (B) forms a covalent bond with the ThDP cofactor in the *Pf*BAL (E) active site. Starting from this first intermediate, the pathway branches into two separate reactions, depending on the second substrate: self-carboligation occurs if a second benzaldehyde molecule binds to the enzyme. The resulting (*R*)-benzoin (BB) is regarded as a side product in this study. In the cross-carboligation reaction, propanal (A) acts as the acceptor substrate, leading to the desired product (*R*)-2-hydroxy-1-phenylbutan-1-one (BA). Both the self-carboligation and the cross-carboligation are modeled as ordered bi-uni reaction mechanisms. The third reaction pathway describes the transfer reaction between the two carboligation products and is modeled as a ping-pong-bi-bi mechanism.

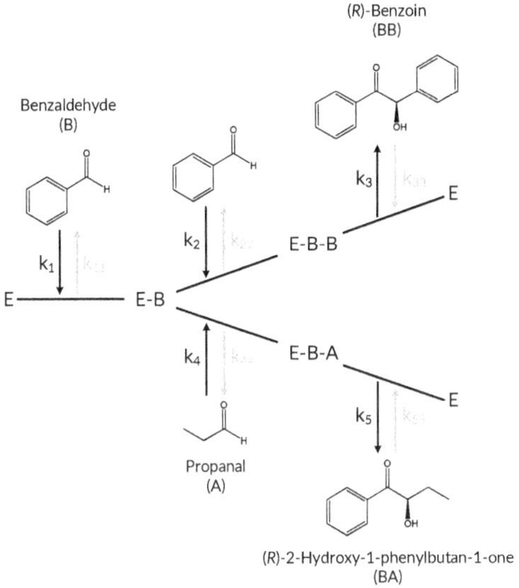

Figure 4.1: Branched reaction scheme for *Pf*BAL-catalyzed carboligations with benzaldehyde and propanal as substrates [51].

Intensification cases

In this chapter, different intensification cases were investigated in order to ascertain the best case for the maximization of the final concentration of (*R*)-2-hydroxy-1-phenylbutan-1-one produced from the *Pf*BAL-catalyzed carboligation between propanal and benzaldehyde. First of all, a reference case was chosen to benchmark the performance of other intensification cases on it. A batch reactor was selected as the reference case because it is the most common reactor used for progress curve analysis for enzyme-catalyzed reactions. Due to rapid enzyme inactivation caused by the substrates (propanal and benzaldehyde), it was posited that dosing intensification concepts could be advantageous over the batch reactor. Therefore, three intensification cases involving dosing were considered in a rigorous and systematic manner. In the following, the three cases will be described.

Case 1: Dosing of propanal. In this case, the possibility of dosing propanal during the course of the reaction was considered to see if it leads to improvements in the final concentration of (*R*)-2-hydroxy-1-phenylbutan-1-one in comparison to the reference batch reactor. Here, the dosing (volumetric) flux of A, q_A was dynamically optimized and the dosing flux of B was set to zero ($q_B = 0$). In addition to q_A, $C_{A,0}$, $C_{B,0}$, $C_{E,0}$ and V_0 required for the highest possible concentration of BA were also determined.

Case 2: Dosing of benzaldehyde. In a similar fashion to Case 1, the possibility of dosing only benzaldehyde along the reaction coordinate was investigated. Here, q_B, $C_{A,0}$, $C_{B,0}$, $C_{E,0}$ and V_0 were optimized with the goal of maximizing the final concentration of the target product BA.

Case 3: Dosing of propanal and benzaldehyde. In this work, Case 3 marks the ultimate scenario where all tunable operating conditions are optimized for the sole purpose of maximizing the concentration of (*R*)-2-hydroxy-1-phenylbutan-1-one. In concrete terms, the dynamic dosing fluxes of reactants A and B (q_A and q_B) were optimized to investigate possible interactions between the reactants. Similar to cases 1 and 2, $C_{A,0}$, $C_{B,0}$, $C_{E,0}$ and V_0 were also optimized.

Mathematical model

To carry out a model-based optimization of the reference batch reactor and the intensification cases described in Section 4.2, a mathematical model of the underlying reaction phenomena that includes material and energy fluxes is required. However, in this study, energy balances are not considered due to the mild conditions at which the *Pf*BAL-catalyzed carboligation is performed and the assumption that these conditions are not energy-intensive [137, 199]. Therefore, the kinetic model and material balances are presented in the following sections.

Kinetic model

Key components in model-based reactor design are the reaction kinetics. Here, a detailed kinetic model is used; which consists of equations for the reaction rates for the consumption of propanol and benzaldehyde, the formation of the main product (*R*)-2-hydroxy-1-phenylbutan-1-one and a byproduct (benzoin) and very importantly the rate of inactivation of the *Pf*BAL enzyme. The kinetic model was derived by combining progress curve analysis and optimal experimental design as described in [124, 126]. From hereafter and for ease of notation, the reaction species propanal, benzaldehyde, (*R*)-2-hydroxy-1-phenylbutan-1-one, benzoin and *Pf*BAL enzyme are denoted as A, B, BA, BB and E, respectively. Thus, the reaction rates for A, B, BA, BB and E are given as:

$$r_A = -\frac{N_{BA}}{D} \cdot C_E \tag{4.1}$$

$$r_B = -\frac{2N_{BB} + N_{BA}}{D} \cdot C_E \tag{4.2}$$

$$r_{BA} = \frac{N_{BA}}{D} \cdot C_E \tag{4.3}$$

$$r_{BB} = \frac{N_{BB}}{D} \cdot C_E \tag{4.4}$$

$$r_E = \left(-k_{deact,A} \cdot C_A - k_{deact,B} \cdot C_B - k_{deact,time}\right) C_E \tag{4.5}$$

Note that the reaction rate equations of A and B (r_A and r_B) have a negative sign to denote that they are being consumed during the course of the reaction. For ease of representation, the terms N_{BA}, N_{BB}, and D are defined as the following constitutive equations:

$$\begin{aligned} N_{BA} = {} & k_{22} \cdot k_{33} \cdot k_4 \cdot k_5 \cdot C_A \cdot C_{BB} \\ & - k_2 \cdot k_3 \cdot k_{44} \cdot k_{55} \cdot C_B \cdot C_{BA} \\ & + k_1 \cdot (k_{22} + k_3) \cdot k_4 \cdot k_5 \cdot C_A \cdot C_B \\ & - k_{11} \cdot (k_{22} + k_3) \cdot k_{44} \cdot k_{55} \cdot C_{BA}, \end{aligned} \tag{4.6}$$

$$\begin{aligned} N_{BB} = {} & k_2 \cdot k_3 \cdot k_{44} \cdot k_{55} \cdot C_B \cdot C_{BA} \\ & - k_{22} \cdot k_{33} \cdot k_4 \cdot k_5 \cdot C_A \cdot C_{BB} \\ & + k_1 \cdot k_2 \cdot k_3 \cdot (k_{44} + k_5) \cdot C_B^2 \\ & - k_{11} \cdot k_{22} \cdot k_{33} \cdot (k_{44} + k_5) \cdot C_{BB}, \end{aligned} \tag{4.7}$$

$$
\begin{aligned}
D = & k_{11} \cdot (k_{22} + k_3) \cdot (k_{44} + k_5) \\
& + k_1 \cdot (k_{22} + k_3) \cdot k_4 \cdot C_A \cdot C_B \\
& + (k_{22} + k_3) \cdot k_4 \cdot k_{55} \cdot C_A \cdot C_{BA} \\
& + k_{33} \cdot k_4 \cdot (k_{22} + k_5) \cdot C_A \cdot C_{BB} \\
& + k_1 \cdot k_2 \cdot (k_{44} + k_5) \cdot C_B^2 \\
& + k_2 \cdot (k_3 + k_{44}) \cdot k_{55} \cdot C_B \cdot C_{BA} \\
& + k_2 \cdot k_{33} \cdot (k_{44} + k_5) \cdot C_B \cdot C_{BB} \\
& + (k_{22} + k_3) \cdot k_4 \cdot k_5 \cdot C_A \\
& + k_1 \cdot (k_{22} + k_3) \cdot (k_{44} + k_5) \cdot C_B \\
& + k_2 \cdot k_3 \cdot (k_{44} + k_5) \cdot C_B \\
& + (k_{11} + k_{44}) \cdot (k_{22} + k_3) \cdot k_{55} \cdot C_{BA} \\
& + (k_{11} + k_{22}) \cdot k_{33} \cdot (k_{44} + k_5) \cdot C_{BB}.
\end{aligned} \tag{4.8}
$$

All the kinetic parameters in Eqs. 4.6-4.8 are given in Table 4.1.

Material balances

To ensure that the amount of participating species are correctly balanced during the design process, a dynamic model consisting of the material balances for species A, B, BA, BB, and E is required. Here, instead of using the mole balances as typically done in the EPF approach, it was found that transforming from a molar to a concentration basis led to lesser numerical issues during the optimization. Therefore, the concentration balances for the reactants A and B which are dosed during the course of the reaction are defined as:

$$
\frac{dC_A}{dt} = s_A \frac{j_A}{V} - \frac{C_A}{V}(q_A + q_B) + r_A, \tag{4.9}
$$

$$\frac{dC_B}{dt} = s_B\frac{j_B}{V} - \frac{C_B}{V}(q_A + q_B) + r_B\,, \tag{4.10}$$

where

$$j_A = q_A C_A^{\text{in}}\,, \tag{4.11}$$

$$j_B = q_B C_B^{\text{in}}\,, \tag{4.12}$$

$$C_A^{\text{in}} = \frac{1000 \times 810}{58.08}\ \text{mmol}^{-1}\text{L}\,, \tag{4.13}$$

and

$$C_B^{\text{in}} = \frac{1000 \times 1040}{106.121}\ \text{mmol}^{-1}\text{L}\,. \tag{4.14}$$

Please note that the variables C_A, C_B, j_A, j_B, q_A, q_B and V are all time-varying, but for the sake of readability the time-varying argument is omitted. This also holds for variables C_{BA}, C_{BB}, and C_E in the following paragraphs. In Eqs. 4.9 and 4.10, the left-hand side of the equation represents the accumulation of the amounts of A and B with time, respectively. The first term on the right-hand side represents the rate of dosing of either A and B, and it consists of a binary term (s_A or s_B) and the time-varying molar dosing fluxes (j_A or j_B).

The binary variables (s_A and s_B) take a value of 0 or 1 depending on which intensification case that is being considered. For example, s_A and s_B will both take values of zero if the batch reference case reactor is considered as no reactants are dosed in this scenario. Similarly, s_A and s_B will take values of 1 and 0, respectively for the case where only propanal (A) is dosed along the reaction coordinate. With these binary variables, all relevant scenarios can be easily specified. The last term on the right-hand side of the concentration balances for A and B consists of the rate of the consumption of the reactants propanal (A) and benzaldehyde (B) due to the reaction. Eqs. (4.13) and (4.14) define the values for C_A^{in} and C_B^{in} which are the inlet feed concentrations of propanal and benzaldehyde, respectively. In this work, C_A^{in} and C_B^{in} are set to their pure concentrations based on calculations involving the densities and molecular weights of A and B (see Eqs. (4.13) and (4.14)).

Similarly, the material balances for the products BA and BB, and the enzyme E are defined as:

$$\frac{dC_{BA}}{dt} = -\frac{C_{BA}}{V}(q_A + q_B) + r_{BA}, \tag{4.15}$$

$$\frac{dC_{BB}}{dt} = -\frac{C_{BB}}{V}(q_A + q_B) + r_{BB}, \tag{4.16}$$

$$\frac{dC_E}{dt} = -\frac{C_E}{V}(q_A + q_B) + r_E. \tag{4.17}$$

For the concentration balances for BA, BB and E, it can be observed that there are no dosing terms since the dosing of either the products or enzyme were not considered as intensification cases. Finally, the change in volume with time due to the amount of A and B added during the reaction is defined to ensure that correct volume change is calculated:

$$\frac{dV}{dt} = s_A \cdot u_A + s_B \cdot u_B. \tag{4.18}$$

The volumetric change (Eq. 4.18) is the sum of the volumetric flow rates of A and B (u_A and u_B) considered in each intensification scenario. Here again, the binary variables s_A and s_B previously described help in selecting which particular intensification case is considered. Of specific consideration is the batch reference reactor case where $s_A = s_B = 0$; thus, implying that the volume is constant because $dV/dt = 0$. In this study, the constant volume implication is correct because it is assumed that there is no significant density change due to the aqueous phase mild conditions typically applied in enzyme catalysis.

Dynamic optimization

Here, the mathematical optimization problem required to maximize the final concentration of BA with respect to the material balances is formulated. The generic dynamic optimization formulation for the various intensification problem is defined as:

$$\begin{aligned}
\underset{j_A(t),\, j_B(t),\, C_{A0},\, C_{B0},\, C_{E0},\, V_0}{\text{maximize}} \quad & C_{BA}(t_f) && (4.19a)\\
\text{subject to} \quad & \text{Material balances : Eqs. } 4.9 - 4.17, && (4.19b)\\
& \text{Volume balance : Eq. } 4.18, && (4.19c)\\
& \text{Reaction kinetics : Eqs. } 4.1 - 4.8, && (4.19d)\\
& 0 \leq u_i(t) \leq 0.1 \text{ L/ min}, \quad \text{for all } i \text{ in } \{A, B\}, && (4.19e)\\
& 0 \leq V_0 \leq 3 \times 10^{-2} \text{ L}, && (4.19f)\\
& 0 \leq V(t) \leq 3 \times 10^{-2} \text{ L}, && (4.19g)\\
& 0 \leq C_{i,0} \leq C_{i,0}^{UB}, \quad \text{for all } i \text{ in } \{A, B, BB, E\}, && (4.19h)\\
& 0 \leq C_i(t) \leq C_i^{UB}, \quad \text{for all } i \text{ in } \{A, B, BB, E\}, && (4.19i)\\
& C_{A,0}^{UB} = C_A^{UB} = 100 \text{ mmol/L}, && (4.19j)\\
& C_{B,0}^{UB} = C_B^{UB} = 149.35 \text{ mmol/L}, && (4.19k)\\
& C_{BB,0}^{UB} = C_{BB}^{UB} = 2.78 \text{ mmol/L}, && (4.19l)\\
& C_{E,0}^{UB} = C_E^{UB} = \frac{50}{\text{Mwt}_E} = 8.4862 \times 10^{-4} \text{ mmol/L}, && (4.19m)\\
& t_f = 180 \text{ min}, && (4.19n)
\end{aligned}$$

where Mwt_E is the molecular weight of the *Pf*BAL enzyme which is equal to 58919 g/mol. Eqs. (4.19f) and (4.19g) represent the bounds on the initial volume V_0 and time-varying volume $V(t)$. Specifically, the upper bounds on V_0 and $V(t)$ are both set to 3×10^{-2} L which is the maximum volume of the reactor used for experimental validation. This is done to ensure consistency of both numerical optimization and experimental results.

Eqs. (4.19h) and (4.19i) are inequality constraints representing the bounds for the initial concentrations $C_{i,0}$ and time-varying concentrations $C_i(t)$, respectively. Following this, the upper bounds for the initial concentrations and time-varying concentrations of propanal and the enzyme were set to their respective maximum values used when estimating the kinetic parameters (cf. Eqs. (4.19j) and (4.19m)). This was done to ensure that the kinetic model is valid during the numerical optimization. Also, the upper bounds for the initial concentration and time-varying concentrations of B and BB were set to their solubility limits as represented in Eqs. (4.19k) and (4.19l), respectively. The upper bounds of the solubility limit avoid issues with precipitation during the reaction. Lastly, the final time t_f was set to 180 min for experimental validations.

Implementation

The dynamic optimization problem for each case as shown in Eq. (4.19) was solved by using the direct simultaneous approach as described in Chapter 2. The NLP problem for each case was implemented in the Matlab version of CasADi 3.4.0, a framework for automatic differentiation and numerical optimization [3]. Furthermore, 50 finite elements and three collocation points were used to discretize the dynamic optimization problems for all intensification cases considered; and the resulting NLP was solved by using IPOPT, an interior point solver designed for large-scale NLPs [191] in combination with the sparse symmetric linear solver MA57 [45] from the Harwell Subroutine Library [75]. All computations were performed on a Linux computer running a CentOS 7 operating system with an Intel(R) Core(TM) i7–4789 processor at 3.60 GHz, and 16 GB RAM.

4.3 RESULTS AND DISCUSSION

In this section, results for the model-based optimization and experimental validation for optimal reactor design will be presented.

First, the results for the batch reactor reference case is discussed. Next, the optimization results for the intensification cases—described in Section 4.2—are presented and compared with the reference scenario. The predicted final BA concentration for all cases are summarized in Table 4.2. Finally, experimental validation for the best intensification case is presented in Section 4.3; thus, validating the benefits of applying the EPF-based approach presented in this work to enzyme-catalyzed processes.

Table 4.1: Reaction kinetic rate constants

Rate constant	Value	Unit
k_1	6184	$\mathrm{mmol^{-1}\,L\,min^{-1}}$
k_{11}	93.2	$\mathrm{min^{-1}}$
k_2	68621	$\mathrm{mmol^{-1}\,L\,min^{-1}}$
k_{22}	7294883	$\mathrm{min^{-1}}$
k_3	15955	$\mathrm{min^{-1}}$
k_{33}	26158	$\mathrm{mmol^{-1}\,L\,min^{-1}}$
k_4	1.83	$\mathrm{mmol^{-1}\,L\,min^{-1}}$
k_{44}	0.00190	$\mathrm{min^{-1}}$
k_5	41610	$\mathrm{min^{-1}}$
k_{55}	373	$\mathrm{mmol^{-1}\,L\,min^{-1}}$
$k_{\text{deact,A}}$	0.000157	$\mathrm{mmol^{-1}\,L\,min^{-1}}$
$k_{\text{deact,B}}$	0.00246	$\mathrm{mmol^{-1}\,L\,min^{-1}}$
$k_{\text{deact,time}}$	0.00400	$\mathrm{min^{1}}$

Table 4.2: Summary of optimization results: final BA concentration, $C_{BA}(t_f)$ for each intensification case, where A and B represent propanal and benzaldehyde, respectively.

Case	Dose A	Dose B	$C_{\text{BA}}(t_{\text{f}})$ [$\mathrm{mmol\,L^{-1}}$]
Reference case	✗	✗	5.83
Case 1	✓	✗	5.88
Case 2	✗	✓	6.52
Case 3	✓	✓	6.59

Reference case: batch reactor

Firstly, the concentration profiles of the optimized batch reactor as shown in Fig. 4.2 will be analyzed. For better readability, concentrations of A and E are displayed on the second y-axis and indicated by arrows. The optimal initial concentrations for A and B in this case are 100 and 5.94 $\mathrm{mmol\,L^{-1}}$, respectively, while that of E is 50 $\mathrm{\mu g\,mL^{-1}}$. Starting with these initial concentrations leads to a final BA concentration of 5.83 $\mathrm{mmol\,L^{-1}}$ (see Table 4.2). To achieve this final BA concentration, Propanal (A) starts at its upper bound concentration of 100 mmol L^{-1} and then decreases gradually to 94.17 mmol L^{-1}. Concurrently, benzaldehyde (B) starts at 5.94 mmol L^{-1} and decreases to 0.11 mmol L^{-1} at a faster rate in comparison to reactant A. It can be seen that the optimal initial concentration of A is higher than that of B. This is logical as the rate equations and material balances reveal a proportional relationship between reactant A and the target product BA. That being said, the rate of decrease of A is slower in comparison to that of B. Reasons for this can be attributed to the fact that the consumption rate of benzaldehyde (B) is higher than that of propanal (A). This can also be seen in reaction scheme 4.1 and in the corresponding rate equations.

Furthermore, the concentration of the enzyme reaches 1.08 µg mL^{-1} at the final time (180 minutes) indicating the inactivation of the *Pf*BAL enzyme (E). This inactivation is mainly caused by the thermal instability of E and the presence of benzaldehyde as shown in the enzyme inactivation kinetics in Eq. (4.5) and Table 4.1 where the rate of inactivation due to benzaldehyde is 15-fold than that of propanal. Moreover, it can be seen in Fig. 4.2 that the concentrations of BA and BB reach steady state. Another key observation is that the concentration of BA is somewhat correlated to the consumption of A and B and the inactivation of E. It is also observed that the side product BB decreases as BA decreases. This implies that the consumption of BB also leads to an increase in the formation of BA.

Case 1: Dosing of propanal

With the results of the batch case delineated, the effect of dosing propanal (A) along the reaction coordinate will now be discussed. The optimal initial concentrations for A, B, and E in this case are 100 and 6.00 mmol L^{-1} and 50 µg mL^{-1}, respectively. By dosing A, a final BA concentration of 5.88 mmol L^{-1} is achieved (cf. Table 4.2). This is a marginal improvement over the reference batch case; i.e., a 0.86 % increase of BA. In Fig. 4.3a, it can be observed that the concentration profile of reactant A remains at a constant value of 100 mmol L^{-1} throughout the course of the reaction. This is due to the fact that propanal

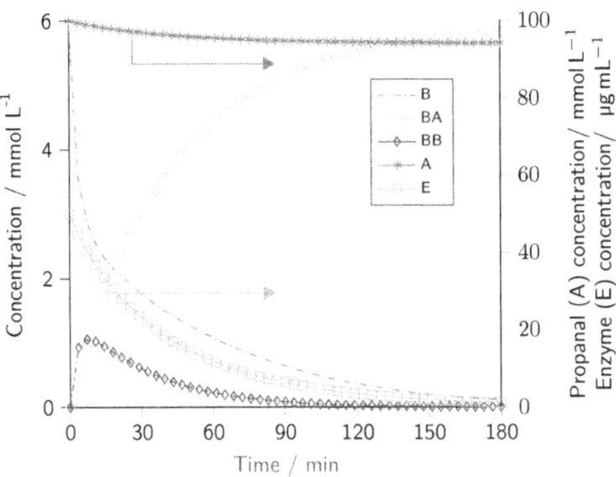

Figure 4.2: Dynamic optimization results for the reference batch reactor case: concentration profiles.

is dosed at an exponentially decreasing rate along the reaction coordinate; see Fig. 4.3b. The constant concentration of A at the upper bound defined in Eq. (4.19j) shows that an increased reaction rate towards BA outweighs the enzyme inactivation caused by A. Setting the upper bound to a higher value might further increase the concentration of BA. However, due to the design space limit of 100 mmol L^{-1} during parameter estimation, the upper bound was kept at this value for the case of validity in this study. Except for the concentration of A, all other concentration profiles are similar to that of the reference batch case (cf. Fig. 4.2). Therefore, it can be concluded that the increase in the final concentration of BA for this case is essentially due to the constant concentration of A. However, this increase in the concentration of BA is only marginal and therefore suggests that the reference batch reactor could be used in lieu of the intensification case where only A is dosed.

Case 2: Dosing of benzaldehyde

The results of the intensification case of dosing benzaldehyde (B) only (Case 2) are shown in Fig. 4.4. The optimal initial concentrations for A and B for Case 2 are 100 and 0.71 mmol L^{-1}, respectively and 50 µg mL^{-1} for E. By considering the concentration profiles in Fig. 4.4a, it can be observed that the profile for A is similar to that of the reference batch case. This

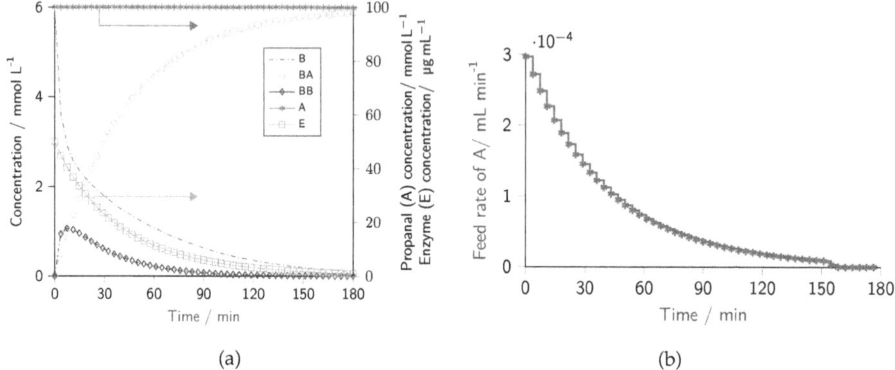

Figure 4.3: Dynamic optimization results for the intensification case involving the dosing of propanal: concentration profiles (a) and the volumetric flow rate of propanal (b).

could be attributed to the fact the that A is not dosed in this case as opposed to Case 1 where only A is dosed.

Moreover, the final concentration of BA observed for Case 2 is 6.52 mmol L^{-1} (see Table 4.2). This is an 11.84 % increase over that of the reference case and significantly better than the final BA concentration for Case 1. By analyzing Fig. 4.4a, this increase could be attributed to the observation that just the right amount of B is dosed (cf. Fig. 4.4b) to drive the cross-carboligation pathway to maximize the formation of BA. This dosing strategy also ensures that fewer reactants and enzyme are diverted to the self-carboligation pathway, thereby ensuring that the competing side product BB is formed at relatively low concentrations.

Furthermore, the initial concentration of reactant B is an order of magnitude lower than that of the reference batch case and Case 1. It can also be observed that the concentration of B remains almost constant but at low values throughout the course of the reaction; see Fig. 4.4a. On the one hand, this almost constant concentration trend is due to the dosing rate of B; see Fig. 4.4b. On the other hand, the general low concentration of B keeps the inactivation of the enzyme due to B to a minimal. Thus, a low concentration of B at each time point also leads to the maximization of the final BA concentration.

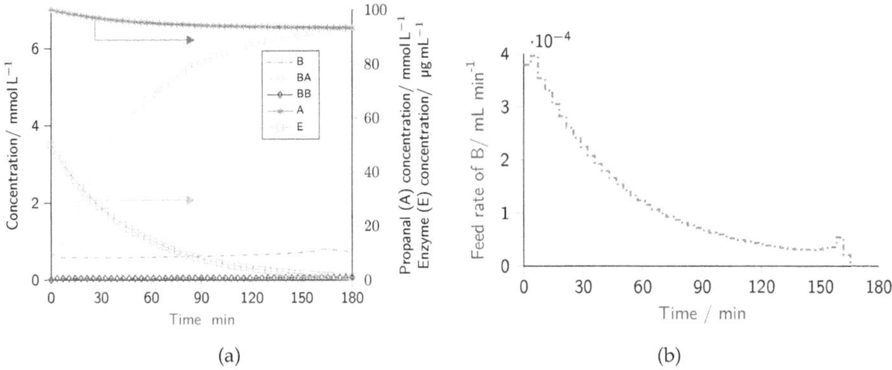

Figure 4.4: Dynamic optimization results for the intensification case involving the dosing of benzaldehyde: concentration profiles (a) and the volumetric flow rate of benzaldehyde (b).

Case 3: Dosing of propanal and benzaldehyde

The results for the case of dosing propanal (A) and benzaldehyde (B) are shown in Fig. 4.5. The optimal initial concentrations for A and B in this case are 100 and 0.70 $\mathrm{mmol\,L^{-1}}$, respectively, while that of E is 50 $\mathrm{\mu g\,mL^{-1}}$. The final concentration of BA by the simultaneous dosing A and B was obtained as 6.59 $\mathrm{mmol\,L^{-1}}$ (cf. Table 4.2). This is a 13.04 % increase over the reference batch case, and it is slightly higher than the value obtained for Case 2. Therefore, it can be concluded that dosing B plays an essential role in maximizing the final concentration of BA.

By taking a closer look at Fig. 4.5, it can be observed that dosing A and B combines the merits of cases 1 and 2. In fact, it can be considered as a superposition of both cases. Hence, the discussions for cases 1 and 2 also apply here; see Sections 4.3 and 4.3.

That being said, dosing both A and B simultaneously leads to the highest final BA concentration from amongst the intensification cases considered. Therefore, dosing propanal (A) and benzaldehyde (B) is the best intensification strategy amongst all cases considered in this work and is selected for experimental validation in the next section.

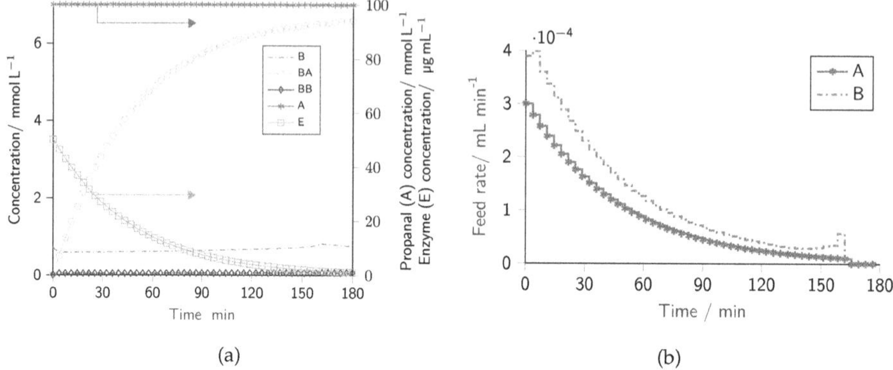

Figure 4.5: Dynamic optimization results for the intensification case involving the dosing of propanal and benzaldehyde: concentration profiles (a) and the volumetric flow rates of propanal and benzaldehyde (b).

Experimental validation

The experimental validations were performed by Dominik Hertwig from Prof. Dr.-Ing. Antje Spiess' group. Details of the experimental set-up and how the experiments were performed can be found in a joint work with Prof. Dr.-Ing. Antje Spiess' group [51]. Nevertheless, the key results of the experimental validation will be presented in this section. Specifically, the results for the experimental validation of the batch reactor and best intensification case will be presented. In order to compare the experimental results to the model-based predictions, simulations were ran for both cases by using the optimal solutions predicted previously.

Fig. 4.6 shows experimental validation for the optimal batch reference case. Note that the concentration of A was not shown because it has negligible impact on the progress curves due to its presence in high stoichiometric amounts. In general, the model prediction were adequately validated by experiments, eventhough small discrepancies could be observed.

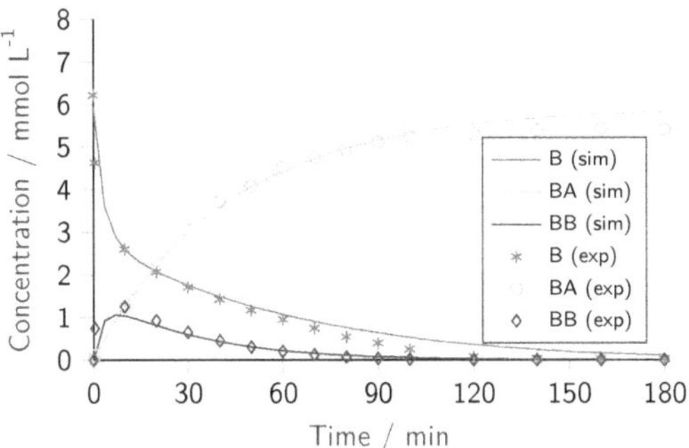

Figure 4.6: Experimental validation for the batch reactor case with the final concentration of BA for the simulation and experiment being 5.83 mmol L^{-1} and 5.40 mmol L^{-1}, respectively.

At initial time point, the concentration of B is 6.23 mmol L^{-1} and is slightly higher than the predicted value of 5.94 mmol L^{-1}. As a result, the experimental values for the concentration of BB are slightly higher than the predicted values for the first 30 min of the reaction. It can also be observed that results of the experiments and model predictions are almost perfectly aligned during the first 60 min of the reaction. After the 60 min, the simulations for B and BA gradually begin to overpredict the experimental values; while the simulated and measured concentrations of BB are closely matched. The joint work with Dominik Hertwig [51] reports that the deviation between the predicted and measured concentrations of B is due to material loss of B during the experiments as a result of excessive stirring, and not due to poor modelling predictions.

Nonetheless, predicted and measured final concentrations of BA, $C_{BA}(t_f)$ is 5.83 and 5.40. This implies that the predicted maximum $C_{BA}(t_f)$ for the batch case is approximately 8% higher than the experimental value—a marginal deviation in this case.

Next, the experimental validation for the intensification case of dosing of A and B is shown in Fig. 4.7. In general, the experimental data confirms the model predictions. The model predictions of BA closely matches its measured concentration or the first 120 min before slight underprediction towards the end of the reaction. The absolute deviation between the measured and predicted $C_{BA}(t_f)$ is approximately 6 %. This slight deviation

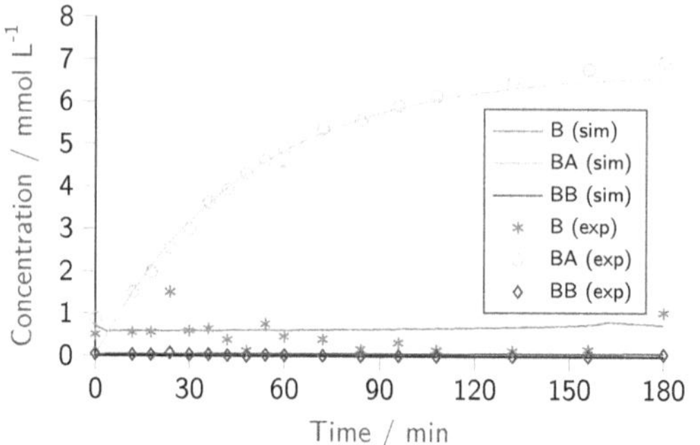

Figure 4.7: Experimental validation for the fed-batch dosing of propanal (A) and benzaldehyde (B) with the final concentration of BA for the simulation and experiment being 6.59 $\mathrm{mmol\,L^{-1}}$ and 6.97 $\mathrm{mmol\,L^{-1}}$, respectively.

could be due to a slower rate of enzyme inactivation in the experiment in comparison to the model [51]. Nevetheless, this is still a good prediction.

In summary, it has been successfully demonstrated and proven that the final concentration of BA after a total runtime of 180 min could be significantly increased by switching from the optimal batch scenario to an optimized fed-batch setup with time-dependent dosing of reactants A and B. This proves that the EPF approach is a powerful approach for designing optimal reactors for enzyme-catalyzed reactions.

4.4 SUMMARY

This chapter presents the elementary process functions (EPF) approach as a viable model-based tool for designing optimal reactors for enzyme-catalyzed reactions. For the *Pf*BAL-catalyzed cross-carboligation of benzaldehyde and propanal, the final concentration of product (*R*)-2-hydroxy-1-phenylbutan-1-one was chosen as the objective function to be optimized.

Following the EPF approach, intensification strategies were analyzed to maximize the objective function. The best results were obtained when both aldehyde reactants were dosed over the reaction time, where dosing benzaldehyde has a more pronounced impact on product concentration than propanal. With the optimal fed-batch design, a 13.04 % increase in the final concentration of (*R*)-2-hydroxy-1-phenylbutan-1-one was achieved in comparison to the optimal batch case. Experimental validations successfully confirm the optimization results.

Furthermore, the apparatus-independent nature of the EPF approach presented in this work could serve as a systematic tool that will enable process engineers to design novel reactors and processes for *Pf*BAL-catalyzed synthesis and other enzyme-catalyzed systems as well. Additional reaction conditions such as temperature, pH value, and composition of the reaction solution can be incorporated in the kinetic model and open up the possibility for further improvements.

Besides optimizing the operating conditions, given the growth of process engineering in developing novel enzymes for API synthesis, it is believed that the results reported in this study can be improved by engineering the *Pf*BAL enzyme. A similar achievement has been seen in enzymes for asymmetric reduction of ketones to alcohols. Biocatalytic process technology has even advanced to a point where reactions such as asymmetric reduction of ketones by biocatalytic routes will outperform the same reaction carried out by competing chemocatalytic methods [99]. By doing this, it might be possible to attain the holy grail of combining protein engineering and process systems engineering [200, 201] in the framework of elementary process functions.

5

ROBUST DYNAMIC OPTIMIZATION OF ENZYME-CATALYZED CARBOLIGATION

Following up on the reactor designs from Chapter 4; which were obtained under the assumption that the parameters are certain, the reactor design problem in the presence of parametric uncertainty will now be considered. Contents of this chapter have been published in [52].

This chapter is structured as follows: in Section 5.1, a brief background about robust optimization and the motivation for the work in this chapter is presented. In Section 5.2, the problem of parametric uncertainties in the *Pf*BAL catalyzed reaction is described. Following this, a novel systematic methodology for robust dynamic optimization is described in Section 5.3. In Sections 5.4 and 5.5, the systematic approach is applied to the *Pf*BAL catalyzed reaction and the results are discussed. Finally, the chapter is summarized in Section 5.6.

5.1 BACKGROUND

Enzyme-catalyzed carboligations need to be appropriately designed, controlled, and optimized. Better designed, controlled, and optimized biocatalytic processes, in turn, will enable environmental compliance, cost-efficiency, and higher productivity. Mathematical models and computer-aided process systems engineering tools can be used to facilitate the comparison of process variants, the control and optimization of processing conditions, thus reducing the cost and time for process development [137, 11].

However, for these models to be of added value for the purposes mentioned above, the models have to be properly calibrated, and the model parameters have to be accurately estimated [206, 124, 161]. A major issue with the accuracy and validity of mathematical models is the presence of uncertainty in the model parameters [178]. Therefore, these uncertainties should be taken into account in the process development and design phase to avoid issues with poorly designed processes during process operations.

To incorporate uncertainties into the design of enzyme-catalyzed processes, [168] advocated the use of uncertainty and sensitivity analysis as good modeling practice for biocatalytic processes. In their work, Monte Carlo simulations were used for uncertainty analysis and propagation. For sensitivity analysis, they advised that the local differential sensitivity analysis method should be used for detailed sensitivity analysis, while the global Standardized Regression Coefficients (SRC) method should be used for checking the effect of input parameters on the model outputs. They also suggested that the so-called Morris screening method should be used only when the SRC results are not reliable.

By using the framework proposed by [168], [140] developed a mechanistic kinetic model for the enzyme-catalyzed transesterification of rapeseed oil in the presence of parametric uncertainties. Although these works [168, 140] have made research contributions in uncertainty analysis, they have not addressed how these processes can be designed to be robust to uncertainty.

To address the latter problem, [116] proposed a systematic model-based framework for optimization of bioprocesses under uncertainty. Their approach involved applying the SRC method to identify the global sensitivity of the system's output to model parameters. Thus, a smaller subset of the model parameters is selected to reduce the computational overhead. Next, stochastic optimization is performed by using a two-loop Monte Carlo sampling method which involves an outer loop where Latin hypercube sampling is used to determine the sample space of the operating conditions and an inner loop where each of the operating conditions is run over the parametric uncertainty by performing Monte Carlo simulations. A key advantage of their work is that global sensitivity analysis can be used to identify key parameters that can give insights into how to better tune and better design enzymes for bioprocesses. However, a possible challenge with their approach is the high computational cost associated with the Monte Carlo simulations and the stochastic optimization step.

Furthermore, a key component of most robust optimization formulations are chance constraints which have to be fulfilled for various stochastic instances. In most cases, these chance constraints are transformed into deterministic expressions by using their means and variances [113, 13]. A common approximation that is used in this regard is the Cantelli-Chebyshev inequality [90, 180]. Even though such approximations have been successfully applied in a number of cases, they do not result in guaranteed bounds for highly nonlinear kinetics and ill-conditioned models that are typically encountered in biocatalysis [13, 130]. An example of such bounds is the mean-variance bound, but for a detailed discussion on the bounds mentioned above, please refer to [13] and references therein.

In order to circumvent such issues, other strategies, such as the back-off strategy, have been shown to be effective [189, 57, 165, 6, 95]. The back-off strategy involves tightening violated constraints and shrinking the feasible region such that the worst-case realization of a given process will still be feasible despite variations in the constraints [165].

Visser *et al.* [189] proposed a fast and robust cascade feedback control strategy for batch processes under uncertainty. In their work, the uncertainties were efficiently handled by using a back-off strategy to calculate adequate margins for the path constraints. By using the back-off strategy, the authors showed that a robust cascade feedback controller significantly outperforms an offline control scheme with re-optimizations.

In [173], an iterative algorithm for robustifying processes by using back-off terms was proposed. This algorithm is initialized by calculating back-off terms from the control inputs of the nominal problem and then iteratively updating the back-offs until a certain convergence criterion is fulfilled.

Another application of the back-off strategy is in the model-based design of experiments (MBDoE). A key paper in this direction is [57] where uncertainty was efficiently handled via time-varying back-offs on relevant constraints during the MBDoE procedure.

Building upon the works of [189] and [173], [165] developed a multistep approach for robust optimization of grade transitions in a polyethylene solution polymerization process in which uncertainties are handled by incorporating back-off constraints. Following the successful application of the multistep back-off algorithm to a detailed large-scale model of an entire flowsheet of the polyethylene polymerization process [165], the approach was used for the robust design of a nonlinear model predictive control (NMPC) algorithm for a two-phase hydroformylation semi-batch reactor [6].

The multistep back-off algorithm [165] has also been applied to the integrated design, control, and scheduling of multiproduct continuous stirred tank reactor (CSTR) systems in the presence of stochastic process disturbances and parametric noise [95]. Although previous studies have considered the use of the back-off strategy for integrated design and control, the work by [95] represents the first attempt to include scheduling as an extra layer of complexity. In their work, two parameters were assumed to be uncertain, namely, the activation energy and the heat of the reaction. In addition to the uncertain parameters, a time-varying stochastic uncertainty in the inlet flow rate (disturbance) to the CSTR was considered. The specific reasons why these parameters were chosen were not mentioned.

As highlighted above, an important component of the back-off strategy are back-off terms which can be defined as (variance-based) margins added to (path) constraints to ensure that these constraints are feasible even in a worst-case setting [189, 173, 165]. Typically, Monte Carlo sampling is used to estimate the means and variances required for these calculating back-off terms. Due to the Weak Law of Large Numbers [14], numerous Monte Carlo samples are typically required to accurately estimate the true means and variances of random variables. Unfortunately, Monte Carlo sampling does not have a good scaling property and consequently, leads to high computational costs especially when dealing with complex nonlinear models like those encountered in biocatalysis.

In this chapter, the point estimate method [159] is proposed as a viable method to reduce this computational overhead. Furthermore, the computational time is reduced by using global sensitivity analysis to identify the parameters that really affect the model output and then propagate the uncertainty of these parameters only. Here, global sensitivity analysis serves as a scientific tool for justifying the relevance of parameters and their uncertainties. Therefore, this chapter presents a systematic, robust optimization framework for the carboligation of propanal and benzaldehyde catalyzed by benzaldehyde lyase from *Pseudomonas fluorescens* (*Pf*BAL) to produce (*R*)-2-hydroxy-1-phenylbutan-1-one.

5.2 PROBLEM DESCRIPTION

As discussed in the introductory section, the robust optimization of a *Pf*BAL-catalyzed carboligation reaction, in the presence of parametric uncertainty, is considered. The reaction mechanism for this reaction is shown in Fig. 4.1. The reactants are propanal (A) and benzaldehyde (B) which are catalyzed by *Pf*BAL (E) to form (*R*)-2-hydroxy-1-phenylbutan-1-one (BA) and benzoin (BB) as the main product and as the side product, respectively. The mathematical model used to describe these reaction pathways was introduced in Section 4.2. Key elements of this model are parameters which have to be accurately estimated to ensure that the model is feasible for the reactor design and process development. Unfortunately, these parameters are uncertain due to imperfect experimental conditions and inherent measurement errors. Therefore, there is a need to determine the optimal profiles and conditions that ensure that the derived reactor design is feasible despite parametric uncertainties.

5.3 METHODOLOGY

The key components of the proposed robust optimization framework is graphically summarized in Fig. 5.1. First, the elementary process function (EPF) approach which was already introduced in Chapter 2 is used to determine the optimal reaction route by considering different intensification cases. The best intensification case (i.e. the optimal reaction route) from the EPF step is then selected and analyzed in more detail. Next, forward realizations of the best intensification case are performed at Monte Carlo (parameter) sample points. This is done to determine which constraints are violated for the different parameter realizations. Once these constraints are determined, the next task is to robustify the violated constraints [141].

Subsequently, global sensitivity analysis is applied to select the relevant parameters that affect the states associated with the constraints which were violated in the previous step. Next, the best intensification case is robustified by using a time-varying back-off strategy. A major novelty of this work is the use of the point estimate method (PEM) instead of Monte Carlo simulations to calculate the statistical moments required for the back-off calculations. As a result, the PEM is briefly described and then followed by a detailed explanation of the PEM-based back-off algorithm. Finally, the root-mean-square error (RMSE) is used to benchmark the accuracy of the approach in comparison to the Monte Carlo–based approach.

Point estimate method

Before demonstrating the robust optimization approach, the point estimate method (PEM) is briefly described. The point estimate method is used instead of Monte Carlo simulations to estimate the statistical moments, i.e. expected values and variances, required to calculate the time-varying back-offs $\mathbf{b}_c(t)$. The PEM approximates the statistical moments of a random variable by using deterministic sample points [101, 159, 204]. The PEM points are

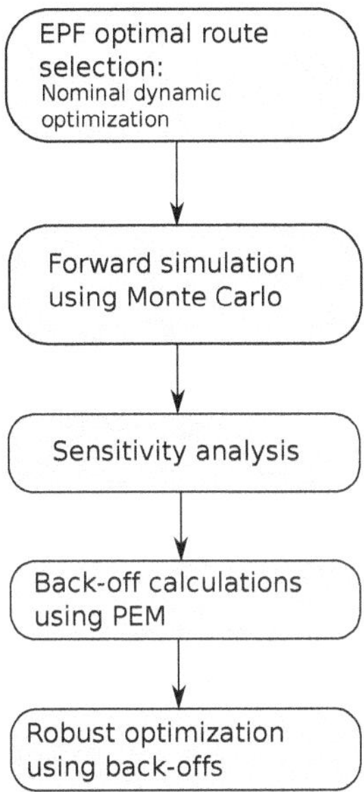

Figure 5.1: Workflow of the robust optimization strategy.

usually fewer than Monte Carlo sample points, but have been shown to reach accuracies close to Monte Carlo simulations even for highly nonlinear systems [159].

In this work, the second-order PEM [159] was used to generate n_p deterministic sample points. The number of PEM points is given as:

$$n_p = 2n_{\xi}^2 + 1, \tag{5.1}$$

where n_{ξ} is the dimension of vector of random variables ξ—which could be a vector of uncertain model parameters as considered in this work.

The PEM points used in computing the statistical moments in this chapter were kindly provided by Xiangzhong Xie and are the exact points used in a joint work [52]. More details on how these points were generated can be found in Reference [52] and the references therein.

As already discussed, the typical robust optimization is more difficult to apply for reactor design problems involving enzyme-catalyzed reactions. This is due to the complex kinetic equations and possible ill-conditioned model equations. As such, the parametric uncertainties are handled by adopting the concept of back-off constraints [173, 165].

For the back-off strategy, the inequality (path) constraints defined in problem (2.3) are firstly considered:

$$\mathbf{h}(\mathbf{x}(t), \mathbf{z}(t), \mathbf{u}(t), \boldsymbol{\theta}) \leq \mathbf{0}. \tag{5.2}$$

Next, it is ensured that the path constraints are fulfilled in the presence of uncertainties by introducing time-varying back-off terms to the constraints at the nominal parameter vector $\bar{\boldsymbol{\theta}}$. Please note that constant back-off terms could also be used. In such a case, the value of the constant back-off terms will be set to the maximum variability (margin) across the time domain. Time-varying back-offs are preferred in this thesis, because they lead to less conservative robust solutions in comparison to constant back-off terms [165, 95]. Therefore, the modified path constraints with time-varying back-offs $\mathbf{b}_c(t) \geq \mathbf{0}$ read as:

$$\mathbf{h}(\mathbf{x}(t), \mathbf{z}(t), \mathbf{u}(t), \bar{\boldsymbol{\theta}}) + \mathbf{b}_c(t) \leq \mathbf{0}. \tag{5.3}$$

Next, the original path constraints (5.2) are replaced with Eq. (5.3) to give a modified dynamic optimization problem with time-varying back-offs as shown below:

$$\begin{aligned}
\underset{\mathbf{x}(\cdot),\mathbf{u}(\cdot),\mathbf{z}(\cdot)}{\text{minimize}} \quad & \Phi(\mathbf{x}(t_f)) \\
\text{subject to} \quad & \dot{\mathbf{x}}(t) = \mathbf{f}(\mathbf{x}(t), \mathbf{z}(t), \mathbf{u}(t), \bar{\boldsymbol{\theta}}), \quad \forall t \in \mathcal{T}, \\
& \mathbf{g}(\mathbf{x}(t), \mathbf{z}(t), \mathbf{u}(t), \bar{\boldsymbol{\theta}}) = \mathbf{0}, \quad \forall t \in \mathcal{T}, \\
& \mathbf{h}(\mathbf{x}(t), \mathbf{z}(t), \mathbf{u}(t), \bar{\boldsymbol{\theta}}) + \mathbf{b}_c(t) \leq \mathbf{0}, \quad \forall t \in \mathcal{T}, \\
& \mathbf{x}(t_0) = \mathbf{x}_0, \\
& \mathbf{u}(t) \in \mathcal{U},
\end{aligned} \tag{5.4}$$

on the time horizon $\mathcal{T} := [t_0, t_f] \subset \mathbb{R}$.

Here, the subscript $c \in [0,\ 1]$ in the back-offs terms $\mathbf{b}_c(t)$ defines the confidence level of the robust solution as the probability that the jth inequality constraint h_j is satisfied in the presence of uncertainty, $c = \mathbb{P}[h_j(\mathbf{x}(t), \mathbf{z}(t), \mathbf{u}(t), \boldsymbol{\theta}) \leq 0]$. For example, a confidence level of $c = 0.99$ implies that the constraint h_j should be fulfilled for 99 % of the scenarios.

Furthermore, the back-off terms $\mathbf{b}_c(t)$ are assumed to be insensitive to the decision variables [165]. Here, this assumption is justified as the back-off algorithm presented in Section 5.3 terminates after one iteration. Under this assumption, it has been proven by [165] that the back-off formulation (5.4) is equivalent to a multi-scenario problem [42] with the Karush-Kuhn-Tucker (KKT) conditions defined at a set of critical uncertainty points where path constraints are active. Please see [165] for more details.

PEM-based back-off algorithm

The PEM-based back-off algorithm is presented in Algorithm 1. The main steps of the algorithm are explained as follows:

1. First, the algorithm is initialized by setting the back-offs for constraint j at all collocation points in finite elements to zero; i.e., $\mathbf{b}^j_{\mathrm{c,pem}}(t) = 0$. The iteration counter is set to $m = 0$, and the maximum number of iterations $m_{\max}$ is set. The PEM points are selected as described in Section 5.3, the parameter η determining the confidence level is set, and the tolerances $\epsilon^{\Phi}_{\mathrm{tol}}$ and $\epsilon^{\mathrm{rmse}}_{\mathrm{tol}}$ for the convergence of the algorithm are set. For the problem considerd in this chapter, it is recommended to set both $\epsilon^{\Phi}_{\mathrm{tol}}$ and $\epsilon^{\mathrm{rmse}}_{\mathrm{tol}}$ to a default value of 10^{-2}.

2. Next, the nominal dynamic optimization problem (2.3) is solved at the nominal parameter point $\bar{\boldsymbol{\theta}}$ to obtain the nominal optimal controls $\mathbf{u}^*(t)$, states $\mathbf{x}^*(t)$, $\mathbf{z}^*(t)$, and the objective value $\Phi^*(t_f)$.

3. By using the nominal control trajectories and key decision variables, such as the initial condition, forward simulations of the system are performed for each PEM point to obtain different realizations.

4. Next, the time-varying back-offs are calculated based on the simulation results by using the following equations:

$$\mathbf{b}^{j}_{c,\text{pem}}(t) = \eta \times \sqrt{\mathbb{V}[\mathbf{h}_j(t)]} \tag{5.5}$$

$$\begin{aligned}\mathbb{E}[\mathbf{h}_j(t)] = w_0\mathbf{h}_j(t, \text{GF}[0]) + w_1 \sum \mathbf{h}_j(t, \text{GF}[\pm\vartheta]) + \\ w_2 \sum \mathbf{h}_j(t, \text{GF}[\pm\vartheta, \pm\vartheta])\end{aligned} \tag{5.6}$$

$$\begin{aligned}\mathbb{V}[\mathbf{h}_j(t)] = {} & w_0(\mathbf{h}_j(t, \text{GF}[0]) - \mathbb{E}[\mathbf{h}_j(t)])^2 \\ & + w_1 \sum (\mathbf{h}_j(t, \text{GF}[\pm\vartheta]) - \mathbb{E}[\mathbf{h}_j(t)])^2 \\ & + w_2 \sum (\mathbf{h}_j(t, \text{GF}[\pm\vartheta, \pm\vartheta]) - \mathbb{E}[\mathbf{h}_j(t)])^2.\end{aligned} \tag{5.7}$$

where η is a tuning parameter determined by the confidence interval c and the distribution of the parametric uncertainty. GF[·] is a PEM-generator function which is defined in [101], and as the name implies is used to generate the PEM sample points. Note that the means and variances at each time point are approximated by using the PEM (cf. Section 5.3).

5. The dynamic optimization problem with the calculated time-varying back-offs (i.e. Eq. (5.4)) is then solved.

6. Next, the counter m is updated, and the difference between the back-offs of the constraint j at the current iteration $\mathbf{b}^{j,m}_{c,\text{pem}}$ and the previous iteration $\mathbf{b}^{j,m-1}_{c,\text{pem}}$ is checked by using the root-mean-square error (RMSE) ϵ^{rmse}. These vectors (back-offs) are of

the same dimension $|\mathcal{T}|$ which is equal to the number of time points at which the back-off values were calculated. In addition, the relative difference ϵ^{Φ} between the expected values of the objective at the current iteration and the previous iteration is determined.

7. Step 6 of the algorithm is repeated within a while loop until the convergence conditions $\epsilon^{\Phi} < \epsilon^{\Phi}_{\text{tol}}$ and $\epsilon^{\text{rmse}} < \epsilon^{\text{rmse}}_{\text{tol}}$ are satisfied or the maximum number of iteration m_{max} is reached, and the algorithm terminates.

8. Lastly, the robust optimal controls and states are obtained and validated with the Monte Carlo-based back-off approach as presented in Section 22.

Assessment of estimation accuracy

To assess the accuracy of the back-offs calculated by using the PEM, the back-off algorithm is also run by using Monte Carlo simulations to calculate the means and variances. Here, the Monte Carlo simulations were used as a benchmark for the PEM since they are assumed to lead to more accurate estimates of the statistical moments due to the Weak Law of Large Numbers [14].

The only difference between the PEM-based back-off algorithm and the Monte Carlo-based back-off algorithm lies in the way that the statistical moments are calculated. In the case of the Monte Carlo approach, the mean and variance of the jth inequality constraint are given by the following natural estimators:

$$\mathbb{E}[\mathbf{h}_j(t)] = \frac{\sum_{i=1}^{N} \mathbf{h}_j(\mathbf{x}(t), \mathbf{z}(t), \mathbf{u}(t), \boldsymbol{\theta}_i)}{N}, \tag{5.8}$$

$$\mathbb{V}[\mathbf{h}_j(t)] = \frac{\sum_{i=1}^{N} (\mathbf{h}_j(\mathbf{x}(t), \mathbf{z}(t), \mathbf{u}(t), \boldsymbol{\theta}_i) - \mathbb{E}[\mathbf{h}_j(t)])^2}{N-1}, \tag{5.9}$$

where N is the number of Monte Carlo samples.

Algorithm 1: Back-off algorithm for robust optimization

Set counter $m = 0$ and $m_{\max}$

Initialize $\mathbf{b}_{c,\text{pem}}^{j,m} \longleftarrow \mathbf{0}$

Choose PEM points as described in [159]

Set n_p from Eq. (5.1)

Set η, $\epsilon_{\text{tol}}^{\Phi}$, $\epsilon_{\text{tol}}^{\text{rmse}}$

Solve the nominal problem (2.3) at $\bar{\boldsymbol{\theta}}$ for $\mathbf{u}^*(t)$, $\mathbf{x}^*(t)$, $\mathbf{z}^*(t)$, $\Phi^*(t_{\text{f}})$

Simulate $\dot{\mathbf{x}}(t) = \mathbf{f}(\mathbf{x}(t), \mathbf{z}(t), \mathbf{u}(t), \boldsymbol{\theta}_p), \quad \forall p \in \{1, \dots, n_p\}$ with $\mathbf{x}^*(0)$, $\mathbf{u}^*(t)$

Update counter $m \longleftarrow m + 1$

Calculate $\mathbf{b}_{c,\text{pem}}^{j,m}$ with the nominal results

Calculate $\epsilon^{\text{rmse}} \longleftarrow \frac{\|\mathbf{b}_{c,\text{pem}}^{j,m}(t) - \mathbf{b}_{c,\text{pem}}^{j,m-1}(t)\|}{\sqrt{|\mathcal{T}|}}$

Calculate $\mathbb{E}[\Phi(\mathbf{x}(t_{\text{f}}))]_m$

Set $\epsilon^{\Phi} \longleftarrow 1$

while $\epsilon^{\Phi} > \epsilon_{\text{tol}}^{\Phi}$ and $\epsilon^{\text{rmse}} > \epsilon_{\text{tol}}^{\text{rmse}}$ and $m < m_{\max}$ **do**

Solve optimization with back-offs (5.4) for $\mathbf{u}^*(t)$, $\mathbf{x}^*(t)$, $\mathbf{z}^*(t)$, $\Phi^*(t_{\text{f}})$

Simulate $\dot{\mathbf{x}}(t) = \mathbf{f}(\mathbf{x}(t), \mathbf{z}(t), \mathbf{u}(t), \boldsymbol{\theta}_p), \quad \forall p \in \{1, \dots, n_p\}$ with $\mathbf{x}^*(0)$, $\mathbf{u}^*(t)$

Update counter $m \longleftarrow m + 1$

Calculate $\mathbf{b}_{c,\text{pem}}^{j,m}$ for the next iteration

Calculate $\epsilon^{\text{rmse}} \longleftarrow \frac{\|\mathbf{b}_{c,\text{pem}}^{j,m}(t) - \mathbf{b}_{c,\text{pem}}^{j,m-1}(t)\|}{\sqrt{|\mathcal{T}|}}$

Calculate $\mathbb{E}[\Phi(\mathbf{x}(t_{\text{f}}))]_m$

Calculate $\epsilon^{\Phi} \longleftarrow \frac{\mathbb{E}[\Phi(\mathbf{x}(t_{\text{f}}))]_m - \mathbb{E}[\Phi(\mathbf{x}(t_{\text{f}}))]_{m-1}}{\mathbb{E}[\Phi(\mathbf{x}(t_{\text{f}}))]_m}$

end while

Return $\mathbf{u}^*(t)$, $\mathbf{x}^*(t)$, $\Phi^*(t_{\text{f}})$

Next, the PEM-based back-offs are compared to the Monte Carlo-based back-offs by using the RMSE [23]:

$$\mathbf{rmse}(\mathbf{b}^j_{c,\mathrm{mc}}(t) - \mathbf{b}^j_{c,\mathrm{pem}}(t)) = \frac{\|\mathbf{b}^j_{c,\mathrm{mc}}(t) - \mathbf{b}^j_{c,\mathrm{pem}}(t)\|}{\sqrt{|T|}}, \tag{5.10}$$

where $\mathbf{b}^j_{c,\mathrm{mc}}$ and $\mathbf{b}^j_{c,\mathrm{pem}}$ are the time-varying back-offs of the constraint j calculated from the Monte Carlo simulations and the PEM, respectively, and $\|\cdot\|$ refers to the Euclidean norm.

Implementation

The nominal and robust dynamic optimization problems were implemented in the Matlab version of CasADi 3.4.0 [3]. Furthermore, 50 finite elements and 3 Radau collocation points were used to discretize the dynamic optimization problems as described in Section 2.3.

The resulting NLP problems were solved by using IPOPT [191] with the MA57 linear solver [45, 75]. The sparsity patterns of Hessian and Jacobian matrices are shown in Appendix B.5 (cf. Fig. B.5). The sparsity and structure of these matrices are advantageous as the IPOPT algorithm is able to exploit this sparsity to solve the NLP faster. All computations were performed on a UNIX-based laptop with a 2.7 GHz Intel Core i5 processor and 8 GB RAM.

5.4 OPTIMIZATION STRATEGIES FOR *pf*BAL-CATALYZED CARBOLIGATION WITHOUT UNCERTAINTIES

In this section, the optimization formulation and results are presented for the case study considered without uncertainties. That is, the nominal problem is analyzed first.

Model formulation

The same material balances introduced in Section 4.2 are used here, but are represented in a state-vector form to be consistent with the notation in this chapter.

Here, the material balances are also presented in concentration basis to ensure the proper and consistent representation of the path constraints which will be shown in the next section. The proper representation of these path constraints is important because a major aim of this work is to ensure that they are not violated due to parametric uncertainty.

$$\dot{\mathbf{x}}(t) = \mathbf{f}_{\mathrm{epf}}(\mathbf{x}(t), \mathbf{z}(t), \mathbf{u}(t), \boldsymbol{\theta}) = \begin{bmatrix} \frac{j_{\mathrm{A}}}{V} - \frac{C_{\mathrm{A}}}{V}(q_{\mathrm{A}} + q_{\mathrm{B}}) + r_{\mathrm{A}} \\ \frac{j_{\mathrm{B}}}{V} - \frac{C_{\mathrm{B}}}{V}(q_{\mathrm{A}} + q_{\mathrm{B}}) + r_{\mathrm{B}} \\ -\frac{C_{\mathrm{BA}}}{V}(q_{\mathrm{A}} + q_{\mathrm{B}}) + r_{\mathrm{BA}} \\ -\frac{C_{\mathrm{BB}}}{V}(q_{\mathrm{A}} + q_{\mathrm{B}}) + r_{\mathrm{BB}} \\ -\frac{C_{\mathrm{E}}}{V}(q_{\mathrm{A}} + q_{\mathrm{B}}) + r_{\mathrm{E}} \\ q_{\mathrm{A}} + q_{\mathrm{B}} \end{bmatrix}, \tag{5.11}$$

with

$$j_{\mathrm{A}} = q_{\mathrm{A}} \cdot C_{\mathrm{A}}^{\mathrm{in}}, \tag{5.12}$$

$$j_{\mathrm{B}} = q_{\mathrm{B}} \cdot C_{\mathrm{B}}^{\mathrm{in}}. \tag{5.13}$$

Eq. (5.11) in combination with the rate equations (4.1) lead to a semi-explicit differential-algebraic equation (DAE) system, where the state vector is given as $\mathbf{x}(t) := [C_{\mathrm{A}}, C_{\mathrm{B}}, C_{\mathrm{BA}}, C_{\mathrm{BB}}, C_{\mathrm{E}}, V]^{\top}$, with C_i denoting the concentration of species i. The controls are given as $\mathbf{u}(t) := [q_{\mathrm{A}}, q_{\mathrm{B}}]^{\top}$, where q_{A} and q_{B} represent the volumetric flow rates of A and B, respectively; and $\mathbf{z}(t) := [r_{\mathrm{A}}, r_{\mathrm{B}}, r_{\mathrm{BA}}, r_{\mathrm{BB}}, r_{\mathrm{E}}]^{\top}$ is a vector of the algebraic variables. Please, note that the rate equations $\mathbf{z}(t)$ are the same equations used in Chapter 4, while the values of the kinetic parameters are from [52]. $C_{\mathrm{A}}^{\mathrm{in}}$ and $C_{\mathrm{B}}^{\mathrm{in}}$ are the inlet feed concentrations of propanal and benzaldehyde, respectively. The inlet feed concentrations of propanal and benzaldehyde are assumed to be pure and are calculated as described in Section 4.2.

Dynamic optimization formulation

The aim of the nominal dynamic optimization problem is to maximize the final concentration of the product BA by optimizing the flow rates q_A and q_B, the initial concentrations of the substrates A and B and the enzyme E, and the initial volume V_0. Thus, the problem-specific dynamic optimization formulation is given as:

$$\underset{\substack{q_A(t),\, q_B(t),\, C_{A0},\\ C_{B0},\, C_{E0},\, V_0}}{\text{minimize}} \quad -C_{BA}(t_f) \tag{5.14a}$$

$$\text{subject to} \quad \dot{\mathbf{x}}(t) = \mathbf{f}_{\text{epf}}(\mathbf{x}(t), \mathbf{z}(t), \mathbf{u}(t), \boldsymbol{\theta}), \quad \forall t \in \mathcal{T}, \tag{5.14b}$$

$$0 \leq \mathbf{x}_0 \leq \mathbf{x}_0^{\text{U}}, \tag{5.14c}$$

$$0 \leq \mathbf{x}(t) \leq \mathbf{x}^{\text{U}}, \quad \forall t \in \mathcal{T}, \tag{5.14d}$$

$$0 \leq \mathbf{u}(t) \leq \mathbf{u}^{\text{U}}, \quad \forall t \in \mathcal{T}, \tag{5.14e}$$

on the time horizon $\mathcal{T} := [t_0, t_f] \subset \mathbb{R}$. Note that in addition to the controls q_A and q_B, the initial conditions of the states $\mathbf{x}_0$ such as the initial volume and concentrations of species i are also considered decision variables. However, the initial concentrations of the products $C_{\text{BA},0}$ and $C_{\text{BB},0}$ are constrained to zero since it is assumed that no product is present at the onset of the reaction. As a result, $C_{\text{BA},0}$ and $C_{\text{BB},0}$ are eliminated as decision variables. Furthermore, $\mathbf{x}_0^{\text{U}} := [C_{\text{A},0}^{\text{U}}, C_{\text{B},0}^{\text{U}}, C_{\text{BA},0}^{\text{U}}, C_{\text{BB},0}^{\text{U}}, C_{\text{E},0}^{\text{U}}, V_0^{\text{U}}]^\top$ is a vector containing the upper bounds for the initial conditions of the states, and the upper bound for the state vector is defined as $\mathbf{x}^{\text{U}} := [C_{\text{A}}^{\text{U}}, C_{\text{B}}^{\text{U}}, C_{\text{BA}}^{\text{U}}, C_{\text{BB}}^{\text{U}}, C_{\text{E}}^{\text{U}}, V^{\text{U}}]^\top$. The actual values of $\mathbf{x}_0^{\text{U}}$ and $\mathbf{x}^{\text{U}}$ are stated in Table 5.1. Please, note that the upper bounds for A, B and E at the initial conditions and during the operation are the same. The upper bounds for B and BB were set to their solubility limits to avoid issues with clogging [66]. The bounds for A and E are ranges at which the kinetic experiments were performed – this is to ensure that the reaction kinetics remain valid during the optimization procedure. Finally, t_f was fixed to 300 min to avoid quenching the reaction before the enzyme was properly inactivated. This is important because the presence of enzyme facilitates the production of BA.

Table 5.1: Upper bounds for the nominal dynamic optimization problem.

Symbol	Value	Unit
$C^U_{A,0}$	100	$mmol^{-1}L$
$C^U_{B,0}$	149.35	$mmol^{-1}L$
$C^U_{BA,0}$	0	$mmol^{-1}L$
$C^U_{BB,0}$	0	$mmol^{-1}L$
$C^U_{E,0}$	50	$mmol^{-1}L$
C^U_{A}	100	$mmol^{-1}L$
C^U_{B}	149.35	$mmol^{-1}L$
C^U_{BA}	10000	$mmol^{-1}L$
C^U_{BB}	2.78	$mmol^{-1}L$
C^U_{E}	50	$\mu g^{-1}mL$
t_f	300	min

Selecting the best intensification case

In this section, the nominal dynamic optimization resuls for the various intensification cases—already defined in Section 4.2—will be discussed and compared. The optimal decision variables and the maximum final concentration of BA for each intensification case are presented in Table 5.2. Table 5.2 shows that the highest final concentration of BA was

Table 5.2: Optimal initial reactant concentrations $C_{A,0}$ and $C_{B,0}$, optimal initial enzyme concentration $C_{E,0}$ and maximum final product concentration $C_{BA}(t_f)$ of each intensification case considered.

Case	$C_{A,0}$ [$mmol^{-1}L$]	$C_{B,0}$ [$mmol^{-1}L$]	$C_{E,0}$ [$\mu g^{-1}mL$]	$C_{BA}(t_f)$ [$mmol^{-1}L$]
Reference (batch)	11.16	6.61	50	3.11
Case 1	3.65	6.51	50	3.18
Case 2	11.94	1.92	50	3.52
Case 3	0.83	3.09	50	3.60

obtained when A and B were dosed simultaneously (Case 3). In line with the proposed robust optimization framework (cf. Fig. 5.1), only Case 3 will be discussed in the following section. For a discussion of the results of Cases 1 and 2 obtained in this chapter, the reader is referred to Appendix B.

Results for Case 3: Dosing of propanal and benzaldehyde

The nominal optimization results for the case in which A and B are dosed simultaneously are shown in Fig. 5.2. It can be seen on Table 5.2, that the optimal initial concentration of B is higher than that of A. This observation is also supported by the initial feeding rates of A and B as shown on Fig 5.2b.

Furthermore, the enzyme concentration starts at the upper bound of 50 $\mu g^{-1} mL$ in order to produce BA as fast as possible and gradually decreases to zero at about 200 minutes signifying the inactivation of the enzyme. After this point, it can be seen in Fig. 5.2a that the concentration of BA and BB reaches steady state. In addition, the concentration of BB eventually hits its maximum value at the end of the reaction time to ensure that BA is maximized.

Moreover, by dosing A and B, the final concentration of BA obtained is 3.60 $mmol\,L^{-1}$ (see Table 5.2). This is the highest final concentration of BA obtained among all the intensification cases considered, i.e., a 15.76 % increase over the reference case. Therefore, this case is selected for robustification in the subsequent sections.

5.5 OPTIMIZATION OF *pf*BAL-CATALYZED CARBOLIGATION UNDER UNCERTAINTIES

Forward propagation of uncertainty with nominal control

In a first step, 2000 Monte Carlo simulations were performed with the initial conditions and flow rates (controls) of the best intensification case (Case 3). Here, 2000 Monte Carlo simulations were found to be sufficient for estimating the statistical moments. As described in

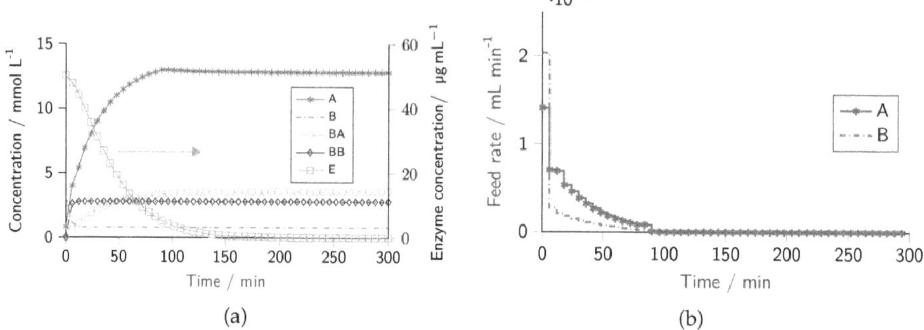

Figure 5.2: Nominal dynamic optimization results for the intensification Case 3 involving the dosing of propanal (A) and benzaldehyde (B). Concentration profiles (states) (a); Feed rates of A and B as controls (b).

Section 5.3, Monte Carlo simulations were performed to determine if the nominal controls led to violations of the upper bounds (see Table 5.1) in the presence of parametric uncertainty. If any of the upper bounds are violated then the subsequent robustification steps (cf. Fig. 5.1) are performed, else the nominal control is sufficient for operating the process. The forward propagation of uncertainty revealed that all the states are within their upper bounds, with the exception of the concentration of benzoin C_{BB}, where the constraint had a 56.95 % of being violated (see Fig. 5.3). Spaghetti plots showing the full propagation of uncertainty for all the states—C_A,C_B, C_{BA}, C_{BB} and C_E—are shown in Appendix B. As only C_{BB} was violated, the focus will be on robustifying C_{BB} by using the PEM-based back-off algorithm described in Section 5.3.

Determining the sensitive parameters

A global sensitivity analysis (GSA) was used to determine the sensitive parameters. The GSA was performed by Xiangzhong Xie and is presented in a joint work [52]. Here, only the key results will be presented. For more details on the implementation of GSA and the results thereof, the reader is referred to Reference [52].

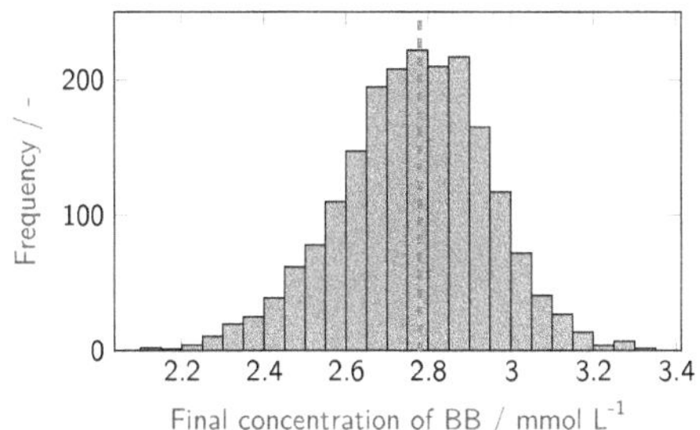

Figure 5.3: Histogram showing the frequency of constraint violation by using the nominal control profiles for the case of dosing A and B (i.e. Case 3). The dotted red line is the upper bound (solubility constraint) for BB.

For the sensitivity analysis, the parameters were assigned normal distributions with a mean equal to their nominal values and a standard deviation equal to 10 % of their nominal values. Results of GSA at different time points for the concentration of component BB are given in Fig. 5.4.

Fig. 5.4 shows that majority of parameter uncertainties have a significant impact on the quantity of interest, i.e., the concentration of BB. However, the sensitivities for uncertainties of the parameters k_{44}, $k_{\mathrm{deact,B}}$ and $k_{\mathrm{deact,time}}$ are negligible, and thus, can be neglected in order to reduce the complexity of the problem. In other words, only the uncertainties of the remaining 10 parameters were taken into account in the following computations. This is important because it reduces the original number of PEM points from $2 \times 13^2 + 1 = 339$ to 201 points—a 40.71 % reduction in the number of PEM points.

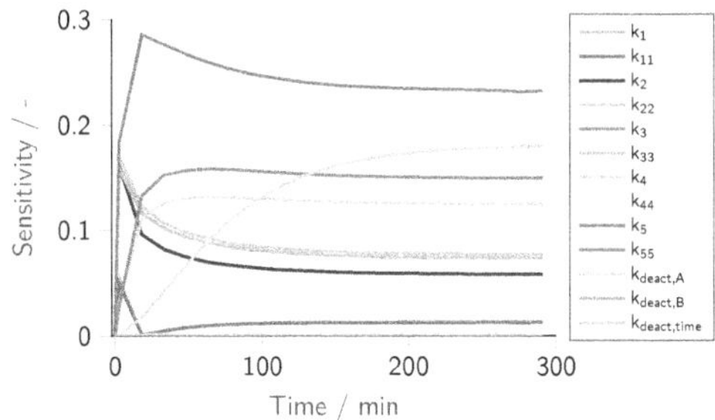

Figure 5.4: Sensitivity results of 13 model parameters for the concentration of BB.

Table 5.3: Reaction kinetic rate parameters [135].

Rate constant	Value	Unit
k_1	597257.2	$\text{mmol}^{-1}\text{L}\,\text{min}^{-1}$
k_{11}	529695	min^{-1}
k_2	1442733	$\text{mmol}^{-1}\text{L}\,\text{min}^{-1}$
k_{22}	22933.2	min^{-1}
k_3	1264217.4	min^{-1}
k_{33}	1988614.8	$\text{mmol}^{-1}\text{L}\,\text{min}^{-1}$
k_4	3273.6	$\text{mmol}^{-1}\text{L}\,\text{min}^{-1}$
k_{44}	13.8	min^{-1}
k_5	568.8	min^{-1}
k_{55}	56886.6	$\text{mmol}^{-1}\text{L}\,\text{min}^{-1}$
$k_{\text{deact,A}}$	0.002448	$\text{mmol}^{-1}\text{L}\,\text{min}^{-1}$
$k_{\text{deact,B}}$	0.001632	$\text{mmol}^{-1}\text{L}\,\text{min}^{-1}$
$k_{\text{deact,time}}$	0.000112	min^{-1}

Robust dynamic optimization formulation

By applying the robust optimization strategy presented in Section 5.3, the back-off dynamic optimization formulation for the *Pf*BAL-catalyzed reaction reads as:

$$\underset{\substack{q_{\text{A}}(t),\, q_{\text{B}}(t),\, C_{\text{A0}},\\ C_{\text{B0}},\, C_{\text{E0}},\, V_0}}{\text{minimize}} \quad -C_{\text{BA}}(t_{\text{f}}) \tag{5.15a}$$

$$\text{subject to} \quad \dot{\mathbf{x}}(t) = \mathbf{f}_{\text{epf}}(\mathbf{x}(t), \mathbf{z}(t), \mathbf{u}(t), \boldsymbol{\theta}), \quad \forall t \in \mathcal{T}, \tag{5.15b}$$

$$0 \leq \mathbf{x}_0 \leq \mathbf{x}_0^{\text{U}}, \tag{5.15c}$$

$$0 \leq C_{\text{BB}}(t) \leq C_{\text{BB}}^{\text{U}} - b_c(t), \quad \forall t \in \mathcal{T}, \tag{5.15d}$$

$$0 \leq C_i(t) \leq C_i^{\text{U}}, \quad \forall i \in \{A, B, BA, E\}, \quad \forall t \in \mathcal{T}, \tag{5.15e}$$

$$0 \leq \mathbf{u}(t) \leq \mathbf{u}^{\text{U}}, \quad \forall t \in \mathcal{T}, \tag{5.15f}$$

on the time horizon $\mathcal{T} := [t_0, t_f] \subset \mathbb{R}$. Note that time-varying back-offs are assigned only to the inequality constraint for C_{BB} in problem (5.15). The reason for this stems from the results of the forward simulations in Section 5.5 which show that only C_{BB} violates its solubility bound and should, therefore, be robustified. By assumming that the parametric uncertainties follow a normal distribution and based on the work of [165], the confidence level c for the back-offs $b_c(t)$ in Eq. (5.15d) was set to 99.9 % by choosing $\eta = 3$ in the back-off algorithm. The tolerances $\epsilon_{\text{tol}}^{\Phi}$ and $\epsilon_{\text{tol}}^{\text{rmse}}$ required for Algorithm 1 to converge were both set to 10^{-2}.

To apply the back-off algorithm, only the 10 parameters identified by the sensitivity analysis to be critical are considered uncertain. These 10 parameters are assigned normal distributions with a mean equal to their nominal values and a standard deviation equal to 10 % of their nominal values. The remaining 3 parameters are considered certain and are fixed to their nominal values (cf. Table 5.3).

Robust optimization results

First, the accuracy of the PEM in calculating the time-varying back-offs is investigated by comparing with the back-offs calculated by Monte Carlo simulations. As shown in Fig. 5.5, the back-off increases with time for both cases; this is attributed to increasing BB concentrations with time, and as such to a decrease in distance to the solubility bound C_{BB}^{U}. As soon as self-carboligation stops towards the end of the reaction, the back-offs stabilize.

Nevertheless, the back-offs calculated with the PEM are approximately equal to those calculated by Monte Carlo simulations from 0 to 80 minutes of the reaction time (cf. Fig. 5.5). After 80 minutes, it can be observed that the back-offs calculated by the PEM gradually become slightly higher than those calculated by Monte Carlo simulations as time progresses. This suggests that the PEM-based back-off strategy could lead to a slightly more conservative robust design in comparison to a Monte Carlo-based back-off strategy. Another reason is that higher back-offs imply higher margins from the solubility limits (path constraints) and a smaller feasible region. Nevertheless, the results show that the back-offs calculated by the PEM are in general very close to those calculated by Monte Carlo simulations (cf. Fig. 5.5). This is further justified by the very small RMS prediction error of 0.0014 as shown in Fig. 5.5.

Fig. 5.6b shows the robust feed rates (controls) for the best intensification case. On a closer look at the robust controls, it can be seen that it follows a similar control sequence like the nominal control (cf. Fig. 4.5b) with some subtle differences. First, the robust propanal (A) control starts at 1.55 $\mathrm{mL\,min^{-1}}$ while the nominal control of A starts lower at approximately 1.41 $\mathrm{mL\,min^{-1}}$. In addition, the robust control sequence for A is coarser than its nominal counterpart within the first 80-minute interval. In contrast, the only difference between the robust and nominal controls for benzaldehyde (B) is that the robust B control starts at 1.95 $\mathrm{mL\,min^{-1}}$ while its nominal counterpart starts at 2.0 $\mathrm{mL\,min^{-1}}$.

In addition to the robust controls, preliminary studies revealed that the initial concentrations of reactants A and B are crucial in ensuring that a feasible solution is obtained for either the nominal or the robust optimization case. As a result, the initial conditions for the reactants and the enzyme were left as decision variables as described in Section 5.4. In Fig. 5.6a, the concentration profiles obtained by using the robust control at the nominal parameter point have the following optimal initial concentrations: 1.07 $\mathrm{mmol\,L^{-1}}$, 2.93 $\mathrm{mmol^{-1}\,L}$ and 50 $\mathrm{\mu g\,mL^{-1}}$ for A, B, and E, respectively. In addition, these robust controls lead to a BA final concentration of 3.47 $\mathrm{mmol\,L^{-1}}$ while ensuring that 99.90 % of the 2000 Monte Carlo simulations are within the solubility limit of BB as shown in Fig. 5.7. However, this comes at the expense of $C_{\mathrm{BA}}(t_{\mathrm{f}})$ which is 3.61 % lower than that obtained for the nominal case as shown in Section 5.4.

As a benchmark, the robust optimization results obtained by using the PEM-based back-off algorithm are compared to those obtained by using the Monte Carlo-based back-off algorithm presented in [95]. As seen on Table 5.4, the 0.10 % constraint violation obtained with the PEM back-off algorithm is very close to the 0.15 % constraint violation obtained by using the Monte Carlo-based back-off algorithm. Furthermore, the final concentrations of BA for the two approaches are almost equal (cf. Table 5.4).

Moreover, using the PEM for the back-off is considerably faster than using Monte Carlo simulations. Specifically, the PEM-based robust optimization has a CPU time of 66 seconds while the Monte Carlo-based back-off algorithm takes approximately 714 seconds. Therefore, the PEM-based algorithm is approximately 11 times faster than the Monte Carlo-based algorithm for the application considered. This speed-up is mainly due to the lower number of PEM sample points ($2 \times 10^2 + 1 = 201$) in comparison to the 2000 Monte Carlo sample points. These results demonstrate that the PEM-based back-off strategy is very efficient and useful for the enzyme-catalyzed carboligation considered in this work.

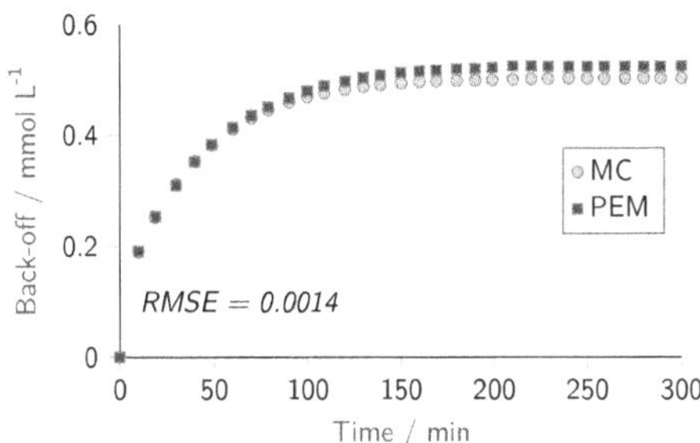

Figure 5.5: Comparison of time-varying back-offs for the constraint $C_{BB}(t) - 2.78 \leq 0$ calculated with the point estimate method (PEM) with those calculated with Monte Carlo simulations. RMSE stands for the root-mean-square error.

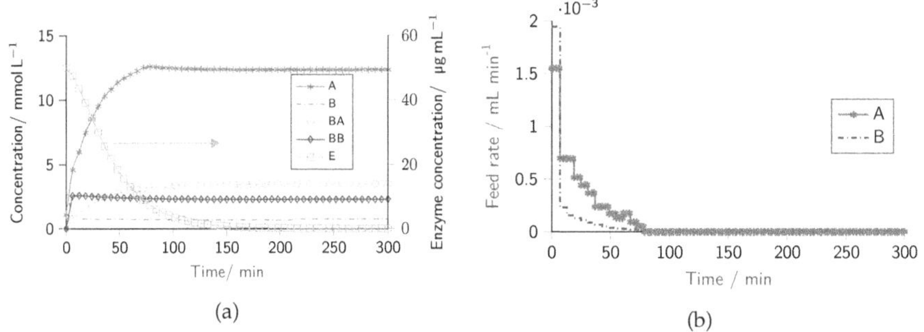

Figure 5.6: Robust dynamic optimization results for the intensification Case 3 involving the dosing of propanal (A) and benzaldehyde (B). Concentration profiles by using the robust control at the nominal parameter point (a); Robust feeding profiles (controls) for A and B (b).

5.6 SUMMARY

A new framework for the robust optimization of enzyme-catalyzed carboligations was presented. The framework ensures that the best intensification case is selected by using the elementary process functions approach and that only critical parameters are considered in the robust optimization step by applying global sensitivity analysis. Specifically, dosing both propanal and benzaldehyde is predicted to lead to a 15 % increase in the final concentration of (*R*)-2-hydroxy-1-phenylbutan-1-one when compared to a reference batch reactor.

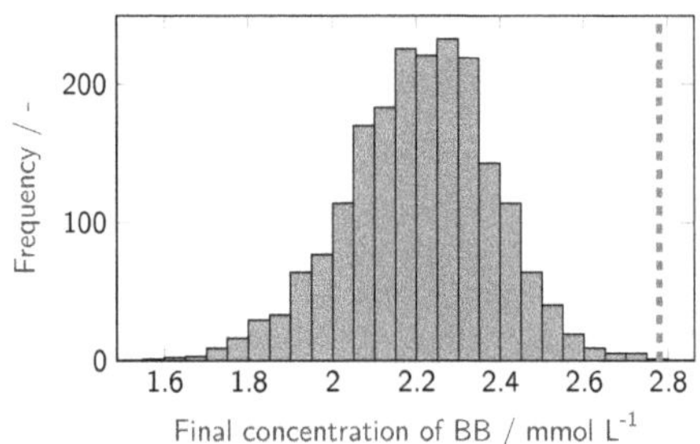

Figure 5.7: Histogram verfiying the effectiveness of the robust control in reducing the probability of constraint violations after performing 2000 Monte Carlo samples by considering all model parameters. The dotted red line is the upper bound (solubility constraint) for BB.

Table 5.4: Comparison of performance of the point estimate method-based (Robust-PEM) with the Monte Carlo-based (Robust-MC) back off algorithm for robust dynamic optimization.

	$C_{BA}(t_f)$ [mmol^{-1}L]	ϵ^{viol} [%]	CPU time [s]
Nominal	3.60	59.56	4
Robust-PEM	3.47	0.10	66
Robust-MC	3.46	0.15	714

$C_{BA}(t_f)$ means the final concentration of BA which is the objective function. ϵ^{viol} means the percentage of constraint violations.

Moreover, a key component of the proposed robust optimization approach is a new point estimate-based back-off algorithm which is shown to be at least an order of magnitude faster than the conventional Monte Carlo-based back-off algorithm. Although the proposed approach does not consider the mean-variance formulation as is typically done in robust optimization, it has been demonstrated that the approach effectively robustifies the reactor design, while ensuring a relatively high concentration of BA under parametric uncertainties.

Another important advantage of the proposed approach is that the dynamic optimization problem(s) within the back-off algorithm can be solved with the same computational complexity as the nominal case. This is easier and more computationally tractable to solve than conventional robust optimization formulations with chance constraints. This implies that the approach presented in this chapter could be easily extended to larger models involving whole (pharmaceutical) process chains. Besides the enzyme-catalyzed carboligation considered in this chapter, the proposed robust optimization approach could be applied to other pharmaceutical processes (and even non-pharmaceutical processes) to ensure Quality by Design.

6

MULTISCALE BIOREACTOR DESIGN BASED ON DYNAMIC FLUX BALANCE ANALYSIS

The previous chapters have focused on the design of reactors on the mesoscale level, i.e. the reactor level, and also on the synthesis of small molecule drugs or organic intermediates. Here, the production of biologics (large molecule drugs) at multiple scales is considered. That is, the reactor design problem is addressed on two scales namely, the microorganism and bioreactor scales.

A novel numerical optimization strategy for dynamic flux balance analysis is also presented. The contents of this chapter have been published in [48] and [49]. This chapter is structured as follows: in Section 6.2, the main features of the model-based approach is described and the solution strategy used in Section 6.3 is presented. Following this, the optimization formulation for the case study considered is introduced in Section 6.4, and the accompanying results are presented in Section 6.5. Lastly, the chapter is summarized in Section 6.6.

6.1 BACKGROUND

The biopharmaceutical industry is the fastest growing sector of the pharmaceutical industry with a steadily increasing market value which attained a total sales value of $140 billion in 2013 and will continue to increase in the near future [2, 193]. This immense growth of the biopharmaceutical industry can be attributed to the potency of biopharmaceuticals, their high specificity, fewer off-target effects, and their effectiveness in treating deadly diseases such as cancer and diabetes [195]. However, the cost of biologic drugs is extremely high and as such makes it difficult for developing countries to gain access to these drugs [105]. A possible solution to this challenge as suggested by [105] is to reduce the cost of manufactured goods (COGs) by increasing product yields while ensuring improved quality and potency per drug amount; this ensures reduced number of doses. Therefore, technological advances in biopharmaceutical manufacturing are required to drive down the COGs. In order to enable such technology advances particularly in fermentation, high-quality host cells and optimal bioreactor design are essential [105, 195].

Typically, an ideal host cell line is one which ensures high cellular growth under economic media requirements, human-like glycosylation patterns, and the ability to efficiently excrete the recombinant protein of interest into the extracellular media [172, 105]. The methylotrophic yeast *Pichia pastoris* fulfills the aforementioned qualities and as such is a popular and intensively studied host cell line since its development in the 1970s [139, 33]. Other features that makes *P. pastoris* a favorable host cell include its tightly regulated alcohol oxidase 1 promoter (pAOX1) and its preference for respiratory over fermentative-based growth; thus, it mitigates the formation of fermentative by-products such as ethanol which could lead to high toxic levels and negatively impact protein expression [139, 32].

Moreover, various strategies have been proposed to improve the productivity of recombinant proteins in *P. pastoris*. These include: intelligent design of expression vectors [172], use of different carbon sources [202], metabolic engineering [156], efficient fermentation protocols [139], and innovative bioreactor designs [117]. Typically, these strategies are investigated by empirical means, but various studies have shown that model-based approaches are key to uncovering strategies that lead to improved production of biopharmaceuticals in *P. pastoris* [80, 41, 39].

Amongst various modeling strategies for *P. pastoris*, first principles dynamic models are important because they predict temporal changes in relevant variables of the bioprocess [28, 156, 121]. Dynamic models for *P. pastoris* fermentation can be classified into unstructured and structured models [106, 183]. Unstructured models are phenomenological models that only consider the extracellular concentrations in a bioreactor and do not take into account the intracellular dynamics of the yeast cells [183, 106]. Nevertheless, they are popular because they can be easily constructed [183]. However, unstructured models are limited because they cannot be extrapolated to operating conditions where there are significant cellular changes [183, 207]. Therefore, they might limit the possibility of identifying novel process windows [68].

Structured models, on the other hand, are more detailed than unstructured models and consider both intracellular information and extracellular conditions [183, 74]. However, most structured models that are available for the recombinant expression of proteins in *P. pastoris* are based on compartmentalized models [121, 119, 30] that do not consider detailed intracellular fluxes.

In contrast to compartmentalized structured models, dynamic flux balance analysis (dFBA) is a structured model concept that predicts changes in the reaction pathways of a microorganism's metabolism due to changes in the external environment in a bioreactor [108, 74]. Several dFBA models have been used to simulate, control, and optimize the expression of proteins in other important microbial systems such as *Escherichia coli* [111] and *Saccharomyces Cerevisiae* [73], but there is a scarcity of dFBA models for *P. pastoris* expression systems.

In an attempt to bridge this gap, [156] developed a dynamic genome-scale metabolic model for the production of recombinant human serum albumin (rHSA) in *P. pastoris*. Their model consists of the dynamic evolution of seven state variables, namely: glucose, biomass, ethanol, arabitol, citrate, pyruvate and the culture volume. They applied the dFBA framework by [157] which involves an iteration between a dynamic block of the aforementioned states, a kinetic block that determines the substrate uptake kinetics, and a metabolic block which determines the flux distributions. However, the work by [156] involves a lot of dFBA simulations to optimize the protein productivity – this could be cumbersome given their iterative approach. Instead, algorithmic optimization could be used to optimize protein productivity by using the dFBA model.

Studies involving model-based algorithmic optimization for recombinant protein production in *P. pastoris* have been reported in the literature. [93] applied dynamic programming to determine the optimal methanol feeding profile for the maximization of rHSA. However, their approach could not predict the product concentrations accurately due to discontinuities in the methanol feed rate. Hence, they used trial-and-error simulations to get an optimal profile that predicts the product concentration – this is cumbersome and could lead to suboptimal results. Moreover, since their approach is based on dynamic programming, it suffers from the "curse of dimensionality" [102, 155] and is unsuitable for large scale problems. Even though the work of [93] represent progress in the use of algorithmic optimization for biopharmaceutical production in *P. pastoris*, they used an unstructured model that does not consider intracellular changes in the yeast cells. Furthermore, [103] combined optimization algorithms, possibility theory, and stoichiometric models to estimate dynamic intracellular fluxes in *P. pastoris*. However, their work was geared towards state estimation and monitoring, and not the maximization of protein production. Therefore, there remains a need for more efficient algorithmic optimization approaches that utilize dFBA models to maximize biopharmaceutical production in *P. pastoris*.

In this chapter, a model-based optimization approach that is based on dFBA for the recombinant production of erythropoietin in *P. pastoris* is presented. As a case study, the production of the glycoprotein erythropoietin [79] by *P. pastoris* growing on glucose is considered. It has been reported that variations in the glycosylation patterns of recombinant erythropoietin can influence its potency [162]. These variations are usually caused by changes in the cell line or process conditions [162]. Therefore, it is important to utilize model-based approaches to predict the effects of process changes before these changes are implemented in the real bioprocess or even before the process is built.

Here, the dFBA model consists of an upper-level problem that is cast within the framework of elementary process functions [56], and a lower-level problem posed as a flux balance analysis (FBA) model [127] – leading to a bilevel optimization problem. Here, the bilevel optimization problem is transformed into a single optimization problem by using the Karush-Kuhn-Tucker (KKT) conditions of the lower-level problem [142]. This transformation is done in order to solve the problem in one-shot without the need for interacting between multiple solvers, i.e., improving computational efficiency [73]. The single optimization problem is a dynamic optimization problem that falls into a class of optimization problems called mathematical programs with equilibrium constraints (MPECs). MPECs present difficulties for state-of-the-art nonlinear programming (NLP) solvers because they violate constraint qualifications required by these solvers [9]. This issue is addressed by using the exact ℓ_1 penalization scheme [9] instead of using mixed integer programming algorithms which are combinatorial in nature [192] or regularization schemes which involve solving relaxed MPECs iteratively [87]. Penalization schemes have been shown to be very efficient for solving MPECs resulting from FBA [205], but to the knowledge of the author, this approach has not been used for MPECs arising from dFBA. Therefore, another contribution of this work is the extension of the penalization technique to handle the complementarity constraints stemming from dFBA bilevel optimization problems. The reformulated optimization problem is then solved at once by using the direct optimization approach [108, 17] and avoids the iterative approach that was previously mentioned [93, 156]. It is shown that the proposed solution approach is fast and efficient, and is able to maximize the productivity of erythropoietin in *P. pastoris*. Fig. 6.1 summarizes the tenets of the methodology employed in this chapter.

6.2 PRELIMINARIES

The dFBA modeling framework is a bilevel optimization problem that consists of an upper-level problem that is cast within the EPF paradigm and a lower-level problem that is mod-

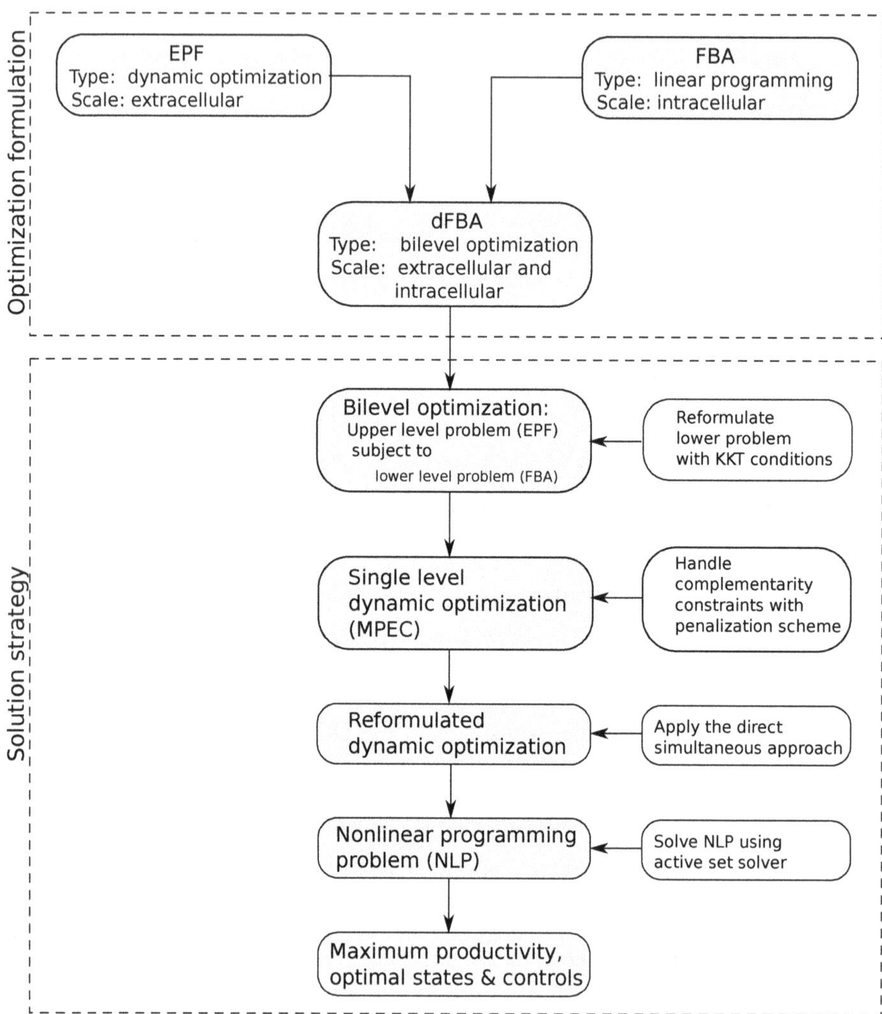

Figure 6.1: Work flow of methodology from the model formulation to the solution strategy. EPF stands for elementary process function, FBA for flux balance analysis, dFBA for dynamic flux balance analysis, and MPEC for mathematical program with equilibrium constraints.

elled as FBA. Therefore, FBA and the EPF framework are described in more detail in the following sections.

Flux balance analysis

FBA is a stoichiometric modeling approach that is used for studying metabolic networks that range from small-scale to genome-scale metabolic reconstructions [127, 21]. FBA computes an optimal distribution of metabolic fluxes within the metabolic network of a microorganism. Thus, it leads to flux distributions that optimize phenotypes, e.g., cellular growth or the production of key metabolites [127].

Before performing FBA, a microorganism's metabolic network has to be represented mathematically by performing what is known as a metabolic reconstruction [181]. This mathematical representation takes the form of a matrix with metabolic reactions and metabolites represented as columns and rows, respectively. The elements of this matrix are the stoichiometric coefficients of each reaction, and as such this matrix is called a stoichiometric matrix [127]. The stoichiometric matrix in combination with a vector representing the fluxes leads to equality constraints that impose bounds on the system. Typically, the microorganism is assumed to be in a pseudo-steady state with respect to the external environment, and as such, there is no accumulation [74].

Next, a phenotype in the form of a biological objective is defined. Typically, the biomass growth is selected as the objective function, but other objectives can also be considered [163, 208]. Subsequently, the objective function is then maximized (or minimized) subject to the aforementioned equality constraints. Unfortunately, the stoichiometric matrix is underdetermined and therefore leads to different solutions that fulfill the same objective [164]. To further constrain the solution space, bounds in the form of inequality constraints are imposed on the fluxes [127]. Therefore, the solution set of these constraints is a convex polyhedron i.e., an intersection of a finite number of half planes and half spaces [22].

In sum, FBA is formulated as a linear programming (LP) problem with the biomass flux as the objective function, a steady-state balance of n (intracellular) fluxes $\mathbf{v}$ through m metabolic reactions, the corresponding stoichiometric matrix $\mathbf{S} \in \mathbb{R}^{m \times n}$, and bounds $\mathbf{v}^{\mathrm{L}}$ and $\mathbf{v}^{\mathrm{U}}$ on the fluxes [127]. It is mathematically expressed as

$$\begin{aligned} \underset{\mathbf{v}}{\text{maximize}} \quad & \mathbf{c}^{\top}\mathbf{v} \\ \text{subject to} \quad & \mathbf{S}\mathbf{v} = \mathbf{0}\,, \\ & \mathbf{v}^{\mathrm{L}} \leq \mathbf{v} \leq \mathbf{v}^{\mathrm{U}}\,, \end{aligned} \tag{6.1}$$

where $\mathbf{c} \in \mathbb{R}^n$ is a weighting vector for the fluxes considered in the objective function, whose elements, in this case, take the value of one for the element corresponding to the biomass flux and zero otherwise.

Elementary process functions representation for biofluid element

In the preceding chapters have demonstrated how to adapt the EPF approach for the design of optimal reactors for the synthesis of small molecule drugs [47, 50]. This chapter takes a first step in extending EPF to the design of optimal bioreactors for the synthesis of biologic drugs [48].

Within the EPF framework, an optimal bioreactor design problem can be formulated in such a way that an extracellular bioreaction functional module is used instead of a bioreactor unit (see Fig. 6.2). This results in the following dynamic optimization problem:

$$\begin{aligned} \underset{\mathbf{j}(t),\mathbf{z}(t)}{\text{minimize}} \quad & \mathcal{J} \\ \text{subject to} \quad & \frac{\mathrm{d}\mathbf{x}}{\mathrm{d}t} = \mathbf{E}(\mathbf{x},\mathbf{z},\boldsymbol{\theta},t)\mathbf{j}(\mathbf{x},\mathbf{z},\boldsymbol{\theta},t)\,, \\ & \mathbf{g}(\mathbf{x},\mathbf{z},\boldsymbol{\theta},t) = \mathbf{0}\,, \\ & \mathbf{h}(\mathbf{x},\mathbf{z},\boldsymbol{\theta},t) \leq \mathbf{0}\,, \\ & \mathbf{x}(t_0) = \mathbf{x}_0\,, \end{aligned} \tag{6.2}$$

on the time interval $\mathcal{T} \in [t_0, t_f] \subset \mathbb{R}$ of the biochemical reaction with time $t \in [t_0, t_f]$, where $\mathcal{J}$ is an objective function of biological relevance, e.g., yield or productivity, $\mathbf{x}(t) \in \mathbb{R}^{n_x}$ is a vector of state variables such as extracellular metabolite concentrations or masses, $\mathbf{z}(t) \in \mathbb{R}^{n_\delta}$ is a vector of algebraic variables such as substrate uptake or growth rates represented by Monod-type kinetics, $\boldsymbol{\theta} \in \mathbb{R}^{n_\cdot}$ is a vector of time independent parameters, $\mathbf{j}(t) \in \mathbb{R}^{n_u}$ is the flux vector containing feeding rates and other key control variables, $\mathbf{E} \in \mathbb{R}^{n_{\text{epf}} \times n_u}$ is the EPF matrix which contains the basis vectors in thermodynamic state space [56], $\mathbf{g} : \mathcal{T} \times \mathbb{R}^{n_x} \times \mathbb{R}^{n_\cdot} \times \mathbb{R}^{n_\delta} \to \mathbb{R}^{n_g}$ is a function vector that defines the equality constraints, $\mathbf{h} : \mathcal{T} \times \mathbb{R}^{n_x} \times \mathbb{R}^{n_\cdot} \times \mathbb{R}^{n_\delta} \to \mathbb{R}^{n_h}$ is the inequality constraint function vector, and $\mathbf{x}_0$ is a vector of initial conditions of the states variables at initial time t_0.

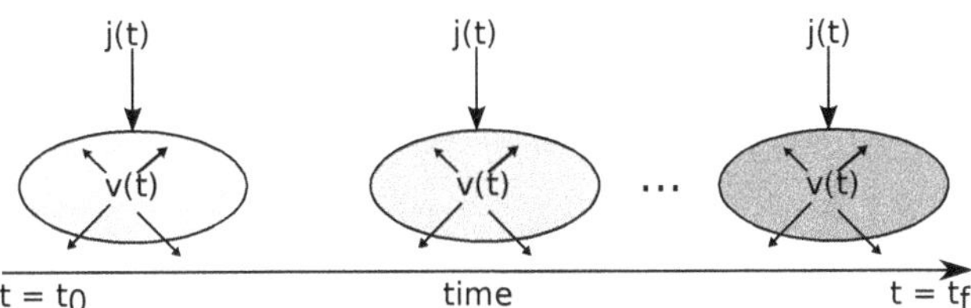

Figure 6.2: Conceptual representation of biofluid element (including cells) in thermodynamic state space acted upon by dynamic fluxes such as the intracellular $v(t)$ and extracellular fluxes $j(t)$.

Dynamic flux balance analysis

The dFBA is formulated as a bilevel optimization problem where the EPF dynamic optimization problem (6.2) is the upper-level problem, and the FBA (6.1) is the lower-level problem:

$$
\begin{aligned}
\underset{\mathbf{j}(t),\mathbf{z}(t),\widetilde{\mathbf{v}}(t)}{\text{minimize}} \quad & \mathcal{J} \\
\text{subject to} \quad & \frac{\mathrm{d}\mathbf{x}}{\mathrm{d}t} = \mathbf{E}(\mathbf{x},\mathbf{z},\boldsymbol{\theta},t)\mathbf{j}(\mathbf{x},\mathbf{z},\widetilde{\mathbf{v}},\boldsymbol{\theta},t)\,, \\
& \mathbf{g}(\mathbf{x},\mathbf{z},\widetilde{\mathbf{v}},\boldsymbol{\theta},t) = \mathbf{0}\,, \\
& \mathbf{h}(\mathbf{x},\mathbf{z},\widetilde{\mathbf{v}},\boldsymbol{\theta},t) \leq \mathbf{0}\,, \\
& \widetilde{\mathbf{v}}(t) \in \underset{\mathbf{v}(t)}{\arg\min} \left\{ -\mathbf{c}^{\top}\mathbf{v}(t) \mid \mathbf{S}\mathbf{v}(t) = \mathbf{0},\, \mathbf{v}^{\mathrm{L}}(t) \leq \mathbf{v}(t) \leq \mathbf{v}^{\mathrm{U}}(t) \right\}, \\
& \mathbf{x}(t_0) = \mathbf{x}_0\,.
\end{aligned}
\tag{6.3}
$$

Here, the rates of extracellular metabolites $\widetilde{\mathbf{v}}$ such as the biomass growth rate and substrate uptake rate are computed by the inner FBA model at each time point. Note that $\widetilde{\mathbf{v}}$ represent the rates (i.e., extracellular fluxes) that are computed by the lower-level FBA and used by the upper-level dynamic optimization problem [74], while $\mathbf{z}(t)$ is the vector of algebraic variables (mostly rates) that are still computed by Monod-type kinetic equations and not by the lower-level FBA. In the next section, the solution strategy (as shown in Fig. 6.1) that is used to solve the dFBA optimization problem efficiently will be presented.

6.3 SOLUTION STRATEGY

Bilevel optimization

In this section, the bilevel optimization problem (Eq. 6.3) is reformulated into a form that is convenient for most dynamic optimization solution strategies by transforming it into a single objective dynamic optimization problem. Moreover, it is also shown how the resulting complementarity constraints are handled.

Karush-Kuhn-Tucker reformulation

Here, the bilevel problem is transformed into a single objective optimization problem by replacing the lower-level FBA problem with its Karush-Kuhn-Tucker (KKT) conditions and complementarity constraints [142]:

$$\underset{\substack{\mathbf{j}(t),\mathbf{z}(t),\mathbf{v}(t),\\ \boldsymbol{\lambda}(t),\boldsymbol{\alpha}^{\mathrm{L}}(t),\boldsymbol{\alpha}^{\mathrm{U}}(t)}}{\text{minimize}} \quad \mathcal{J} \tag{6.4a}$$

$$\text{subject to} \quad \frac{d\mathbf{x}}{dt} = \mathbf{E}(\mathbf{x},\mathbf{z},\boldsymbol{\theta},t)\mathbf{j}(\mathbf{x},\mathbf{z},\mathbf{v},\boldsymbol{\theta},t), \tag{6.4b}$$

$$\mathbf{g}(\mathbf{x},\mathbf{z},\mathbf{v},\boldsymbol{\theta},t) = \mathbf{0}, \tag{6.4c}$$

$$\mathbf{h}(\mathbf{x},\mathbf{z},\mathbf{v},\boldsymbol{\theta},t) \leq \mathbf{0}, \tag{6.4d}$$

$$\nabla_{\mathbf{v}}\mathcal{L} = c + \mathbf{S}^{\top}\boldsymbol{\lambda} + \boldsymbol{\alpha}^{\mathrm{L}} - \boldsymbol{\alpha}^{\mathrm{U}} = \mathbf{0}, \tag{6.4e}$$

$$\nabla_{\lambda}\mathcal{L} = \mathbf{S}\mathbf{v} = \mathbf{0}, \tag{6.4f}$$

$$\text{diag}(\mathbf{v}(t) - \mathbf{v}^{\mathrm{L}}(t))\boldsymbol{\alpha}^{\mathrm{L}}(t) = \mathbf{0}, \tag{6.4g}$$

$$\text{diag}(\mathbf{v}(t) - \mathbf{v}^{\mathrm{U}}(t))\boldsymbol{\alpha}^{\mathrm{U}}(t) = \mathbf{0}, \tag{6.4h}$$

$$\mathbf{x}(t_0) = \mathbf{x}_0, \tag{6.4i}$$

$$\boldsymbol{\alpha}^{\mathrm{L}}(t) \in \mathbb{R}^n, \boldsymbol{\alpha}^{\mathrm{U}}(t) \in \mathbb{R}^n, \boldsymbol{\lambda}(t) \in \mathbb{R}^m \geq \mathbf{0}. \tag{6.4j}$$

where $\mathcal{L}$ is the Lagrangian function given as:

$$\mathcal{L}(\mathbf{v},\boldsymbol{\lambda},\boldsymbol{\alpha}^{\mathrm{L}},\boldsymbol{\alpha}^{\mathrm{U}},t) = -\mathbf{c}^{\top}\mathbf{v} - (\mathbf{S}\mathbf{v})^{\top}\boldsymbol{\lambda} - (\mathbf{v}^{\mathrm{U}} - \mathbf{v})^{\top}\boldsymbol{\alpha}^{\mathrm{U}} - (\mathbf{v} - \mathbf{v}^{\mathrm{L}})^{\top}\boldsymbol{\alpha}^{\mathrm{L}}, \tag{6.5}$$

where $\boldsymbol{\lambda}$ is a vector of Lagrange multipliers corresponding to $\mathbf{S}\mathbf{v} = \mathbf{0}$, $\boldsymbol{\alpha}^{\mathrm{L}}$ and $\boldsymbol{\alpha}^{\mathrm{U}}$ are vectors of Lagrange multipliers associated with the lower and upper bounds of the fluxes $\mathbf{v}$, and $\nabla_{\mathbf{v}}\mathcal{L}$ and $\nabla_{\lambda}\mathcal{L}$ are first derivatives of the Lagrangian with respect to $\mathbf{v}$ and $\boldsymbol{\lambda}$, respectively.

The reformulation (6.4) is valid because the lower-level problem is convex and regular and as such the KKT conditions are sufficient and necessary conditions for optimality [38]. With the occurrence of complementarity constraints (6.4g) and (6.4h), the problem represented by (6.4) falls into the class of problems called mathematical programs with equilibrium constraints [9, 143].

Exact ℓ_1 penalization

For mathematical programs with equilibrium constraints (MPECs), even if the objective function and the solution set of the fluxes $\mathbf{v} \in \mathcal{V}$ are both convex, they are still difficult to solve because of nonconvexities introduced by complementarity and Lagrangian constraints [38, 9]. Moreover, in order to ensure that the replacement of the lower-level problem by its KKT conditions provides a necessary optimality condition, certain constraint qualifications (CQs) such as Guignard's CQ, Mangasarian-Fromovitz CQ and the linear independence CQ have to be fulfilled [190, 97].

Unfortunately, MPECs are known to violate these CQs and as such reformulations are often used to make them tractable for state-of-the-art NLP solvers to handle [9, 143]. Such reformulations can be classified into two main groups namely, regularization and penalization schemes [143, 9]. Regularization involves replacing the complementarity constraints with a constraint that has a positive parameter and then repeatedly solving the NLP as this value is successively decreased to a tolerance that is close to zero [143]. In the case of penalization, the complementarity constraints are transferred to the objective to form a penalty term [143].

In this work, preliminary studies were performed to compare between the regularization and penalization formulations, but the penalization formulation was found to be the most stable for the case study considered in this chapter. Penalization schemes are also favourable because provided that a sufficiently large penalty term is chosen, the reformulated MPEC can be solved efficiently in one-shot. This is in contrast with regularization schemes for dFBA where repeated iterations of relaxed MPECs is required to converge to a local optimal solution [87]. Furthermore, [9] conducted benchmark studies and showed that the usage of well-posed complementarity constraints coupled with the penalty formulation and an active set NLP solver is the most efficient strategy for solving MPECs arising from chemical engineering. This was also the case in this work, and as such, the exact ℓ_1 penalization technique [9] was used in combination with the active set NLP solver CONOPT [44]. The ℓ_1 penalization formulation of (6.4) is given as:

$$\underset{\substack{\mathbf{j}(t),\mathbf{z}(t),\mathbf{v}(t),\\ \boldsymbol{\lambda}(t),\boldsymbol{\alpha}^{\mathrm{L}}(t),\boldsymbol{\alpha}^{\mathrm{U}}(t)}}{\text{minimize}} \quad \mathcal{J} + \rho \left\| \hat{\mathbf{v}}^{\top} \boldsymbol{\alpha} \right\|_1 \tag{6.6a}$$

$$\text{subject to} \quad \frac{d\mathbf{x}}{dt} = \mathbf{E}(\mathbf{x}, \mathbf{z}, \boldsymbol{\theta}, t)\mathbf{j}(\mathbf{x}, \mathbf{z}, \mathbf{v}, \boldsymbol{\theta}, t), \tag{6.6b}$$

$$\mathbf{g}(\mathbf{x}, \mathbf{z}, \mathbf{v}, \boldsymbol{\theta}, t) = \mathbf{0}, \tag{6.6c}$$

$$\mathbf{h}(\mathbf{x}, \mathbf{z}, \mathbf{v}, \boldsymbol{\theta}, t) \leq \mathbf{0}, \tag{6.6d}$$

$$\nabla_{\mathbf{v}} \mathcal{L} = c + \mathbf{S}^{\top} \boldsymbol{\lambda} + \boldsymbol{\alpha}^{\mathrm{L}} - \boldsymbol{\alpha}^{\mathrm{U}} = \mathbf{0}, \tag{6.6e}$$

$$\nabla_{\boldsymbol{\lambda}} \mathcal{L} = \mathbf{S}\mathbf{v} = \mathbf{0}, \tag{6.6f}$$

$$\hat{\mathbf{v}} = \begin{bmatrix} \mathbf{v}(t) - \mathbf{v}^{\mathrm{L}}(t) \\ \mathbf{v}(t) - \mathbf{v}^{\mathrm{U}}(t) \end{bmatrix} \in \mathbb{R}^{2n}, \tag{6.6g}$$

$$\boldsymbol{\alpha} = \begin{bmatrix} \boldsymbol{\alpha}^{\mathrm{L}}(t) \\ \boldsymbol{\alpha}^{\mathrm{U}}(t) \end{bmatrix}, \tag{6.6h}$$

$$\mathbf{x}(t_0) = \mathbf{x}_0, \tag{6.6i}$$

$$\boldsymbol{\alpha} \in \mathbb{R}^{2n}, \boldsymbol{\lambda} \in \mathbb{R}^{m} \geq \mathbf{0}. \tag{6.6j}$$

Here, the variables associated with the complementarity constraints Eq. (6.4g) and Eq. (6.4h) were rearranged into the variables $\hat{\mathbf{v}}$ (6.6g) and $\boldsymbol{\alpha}$ (6.6h). Moreover, the complementarity constraints are transferred from the constraints to the objective function (6.6a) and multiplied by a sufficiently large penalty parameter ρ. The ℓ_1 penalization technique ensures that the complementarity constraints are satisfied provided that $\rho \geq \rho_c$, where ρ_c is a critical penalty parameter [9]. In this work, various values of ρ were compared and $\rho = 10^3$ was found to be sufficient.

Implementation

In this work, the simultaneous approach (see Chapter 2) was applied to transcribe Eq. (6.6) directly into an NLP problem. The extracellular states were discretized on both collocation points and finite elements by using 20 finite elements with 3 Radau collocation points in each element, while the extracellular controls and intracellular fluxes were discretized on the 20 finite elements only by using a piecewise constant parameterization. The resulting NLP was implemented in the algebraic mathematical language AMPL [55] and the CONOPT solver was used [44]. All computations were performed on a Linux machine with an Intel (R) Core (TM) i7-4789 processor at 3.60 GHz, and 16 GB RAM.

6.4 CASE STUDY: RECOMBINANT PROTEIN PRODUCTION IN *pichia pastoris*

As already mentioned, the case study considered is the recombinant production of the biologic drug erythropoietin in *Pichia pastoris* with glucose as the sole carbon source (substrate). Here, the aim is to maximize the productivity of erythropoietin by using the computational approach presented previously. Another aim is to obtain optimal dynamic controls at both the extracellular and intracellular levels that maximize productivity during the fermentation process. The productivity of erythropoietin was chosen as the objective function of the upper-level problem because it is a widely used metric for accessing the economic viability of a bioprocess [4, 174, 96]. Typically, high productivity implies lower operating and capital costs [4].

As a benchmark to compare the optimization results, the experimental work of [29]—in which erythropoietin was produced in *P. pastoris*—was chosen. The maximum concentration of erythropoietin reported by [29] was $130\,\mathrm{mg\,L^{-1}}$ in 24 hours and the maximum working volume was 2 L. Based on these values, the maximum possible productivity obtained by [29] was estimated to be $10.83\,\mathrm{mg\,h^{-1}}$. This productivity was obtained by utilizing the traditional exponential feeding strategy. In this study, no pre-defined feeding strategies were used. Rather, the an optimal feeding strategy (control) was derived by solving the optimization problem.

To model the dynamic intracellular flux distributions, a metabolic flux network adapted from the validated FBA model by [115] was used. It consists of 37 intracellular metabolites and 47 intracellular reactions. The network consists of the TCA cycle, the pentose phosphate pathway (PPP), Embden-Meyerhoff-Parnas (EMP) pathway (i.e. glycolysis), pathways describing the metabolism of methanol, glycerol and glucose substrates, and transport reactions (see Fig. 6.3). In order to consider only glucose as the substrate, the glycerol (flux 43) and methanol (flux 46) uptake fluxes were set to zero by enforcing the constraints $v_{\text{gly}} = 0$ and $v_{\text{meoh}} = 0$, respectively [115, 187]. Note that v_{gly} represents the glycerol uptake flux, while v_{meoh} represents methanol uptake flux. It is also assumed that sufficient oxygen is present for the cells to grow aerobically and as such an oxygen balance is not included in the dFBA model [73].

In contrast to available structured models for *P. pastoris* [119, 121, 30], none of the aforementioned pathways compartmentalized, but all relevant intracellular metabolites and reactions were considered. Moreover, only the first level of EPF was considered, i.e., fluxes such as the substrate feeding rates or dissolved oxygen rate were not constrained to mass or heat transfer limitations. Here, an intensification strategy that involves the intermittent feeding of glucose substrate was considered as the biofluid element progresses in time. This can be physically translated into a fed-batch bioreactor; but, it is considered as a functional module in order to be consistent with the EPF concept [56]. Nevertheless, since the approach presented in this work is based on the EPF framework, it can be extended to other intensification strategies.

Therefore, the following dFBA model is obtained:

$$\underset{\phi(t)_{\text{gluc}},\, \tilde{\mathbf{v}}(t),\, t_{\text{f}}}{\text{minimize}} \quad \mathcal{J} \triangleq -m_{\text{epo}}(t_{\text{f}})/t_{\text{f}}$$

$$\text{subject to} \quad \frac{dm_{\text{biom}}(t)}{dt} = m_{\text{biom}} v_{\text{biom}},$$

$$
\begin{aligned}
&\frac{dm_{\text{gluc}}(t)}{dt} = -m_{\text{biom}} v_{\text{gluc}} + C_{\text{gluc,in}} \phi_{\text{gluc}}, \\
&\frac{dm_{\text{epo}}(t)}{dt} = m_{\text{biom}} v_{\text{epo}}, \\
&\frac{dV(t)}{dt} = \phi_{\text{gluc}}, \\
&\widetilde{\mathbf{v}}(t) \in \underset{\mathbf{v}(t)}{\arg\min} \left\{ -\mathbf{c}^\top \mathbf{v}(t) \mid \mathbf{S}\mathbf{v}(t) = \mathbf{0}, -10^3 \le \mathbf{v}(t) \le 10^3 \right\}, \\
&m_k = C_k V, \quad k \in \{\text{biom}, \text{gluc}, \text{epo}\}, \\
&C_{\text{gluc},0} = 50\,\text{mmol}\,\text{L}^{-1}, \\
&C_{\text{biom},0} = 1.0\,\text{g}\,\text{L}^{-1}, \\
&C_{\text{epo},0} = 0.0\,\text{g}\,\text{L}^{-1}, \\
&V_0 = 0.82\,\text{L}, \\
&C_{\text{gluc,in}} = C_{\text{gluc},0}, \\
&v_{\text{epo}} = a v_{\text{biom}} + b, \\
&m_k \ge 0, \quad k \in \{\text{biom}, \text{gluc}, \text{epo}\}, \\
&m_{\text{biom}} \le 400\,\text{g}, \\
&0.0 \le V \le 3.0\,\text{L}, \\
&0 \le \phi_{\text{gluc}} \le 1.0\,\text{L/h}, \\
&v_{\text{gly}} = 0, v_{\text{meoh}} = 0, \\
&v_{\text{gluc}} \le \frac{\mu_{\text{gluc,max}} C_{\text{gluc}}}{Y_{\text{biom/gluc}}(K_{\text{gluc}} + C_{\text{gluc}})} + \gamma_{\text{gluc}}, \\
&20 \le t_{\text{f}} \le 60\,\text{h}.
\end{aligned}
\tag{6.7}
$$

The presented dFBA optimization problem is then translated into the EPF formulation as follows:

$$\begin{aligned}
\underset{\boldsymbol{\phi}(t),\tilde{\mathbf{v}}(t),t_\mathrm{f}}{\text{minimize}} \quad & \mathcal{J} := -m_\mathrm{epo}(t_\mathrm{f})/t_\mathrm{f} \\
\text{subject to} \quad & \frac{d\mathbf{x}(t)}{dt} = \mathbf{E}(\mathbf{x},\boldsymbol{\theta},t)\mathbf{j}(\boldsymbol{\phi},\tilde{\mathbf{v}},t)\,, \\
& \mathbf{g}(\mathbf{x},\boldsymbol{\phi},\mathbf{v},\boldsymbol{\theta},t) = 0\,, \\
& \mathbf{h}(\mathbf{x},\boldsymbol{\phi},\mathbf{v},\boldsymbol{\theta},t) \leq 0\,, \\
& \mathbf{x}(t_0) = \mathbf{x}_0\,,
\end{aligned} \tag{6.8}$$

where $\mathbf{x} = [m_\mathrm{biom}, m_\mathrm{gluc}, m_\mathrm{epo}, V]^\top$,

$$\mathbf{j} = \left[v_\mathrm{biom}, v_\mathrm{gluc}, v_\mathrm{epo}, \phi_\mathrm{gluc}\right]^\top,$$

$$\mathbf{E} = \begin{bmatrix} m_\mathrm{biom} & 0 & 0 & 0 \\ 0 & -m_\mathrm{biom} & 0 & C_\mathrm{gluc,in} \\ 0 & 0 & m_\mathrm{epo} & 0 \\ 0 & 0 & 0 & 1 \end{bmatrix}$$

where $\mathcal{J}$ is the productivity objective function in $\mathrm{g\,h^{-1}}$, $\mathbf{S} \in \mathbb{R}^{37\times 47}$ is the stoichiometric matrix, $\mathbf{v} \in \mathbb{R}^{47}$ is a vector representing the metabolic reaction fluxes in $\mathrm{mmol\,g^{-1}\,h^{-1}}$, $\mathbf{c} \in \mathbb{R}^{47}$ is the weighting vector as described in Section 6.2; m_biom, m_gluc, and m_epo are masses of the biomass, glucose, and erythropoietin, respectively. Similarly, C_k represents the concentration of component $k \in \{\mathrm{biom}, \mathrm{gluc}, \mathrm{epo}\}$, and $C_{k,0}$ is the initial concentration of component k. $C_\mathrm{gluc,in}$ is the inlet concentration of the fed glucose, V is the volume of the biofluid element, V_0 is the initial condition of the volume at time t_0, and ϕ_gluc is the volumetric feeding flux of glucose.

Furthermore, the glucose uptake flux is bounded by a Monod-type kinetic equation derived from [30]. This is to ensure that the glucose uptake flux at each time point is realistic [108, 74]. For the Monod-type kinetics bounding the glucose uptake flux v_gluc, $\mu_\mathrm{gluc,max}$ represents the maximum specific growth rate on glucose, $Y_\mathrm{biom/gluc}$ represents the biomass-to-glucose yield, K_{gluc} is the glucose saturation constant, and γ_{gluc} denotes the maintenance coefficient based on glucose. The specific erythropoietin production rate v_{epo} was assumed to follow the Luedeking-Piret model [146] and the coefficients a and b were determined by performing a least squares optimization on data from [30] and [103]. For convenience, all kinetic parameters are summarized in Table 6.1. The bounds for final bioreaction time t_{f} and volume V were obtained from [29, 30] and were set between 20 to 60 h and 0.0 to 3.0 L, respectively, in order to ensure a fair comparison to already published results in the literature.

Table 6.1: Model parameters.

Parameter	Value	Unit	Source
a	4.8×10^{-4}	-	This work
b	8×10^{-5}	-	This work
K_{gluc}	0.1	$\text{g}\,\text{L}^{-1}$	[80]
γ_{gluc}	0.025	$\text{g}\,\text{g}^{-1}\,\text{h}^{-1}$	[30]
$\mu_{\text{gluc,max}}$	0.032	h^{-1}	[88]
$Y_{\text{biom/gluc}}$	0.62	$\text{g}\,\text{g}^{-1}$	[88]

6.5 RESULTS AND DISCUSSION

Extracellular states and metabolites

The maximum productivity of erythropoietin obtained after solving the problem in Section 6.4 was 17.97 mg h^{-1}, while the total cultivation time was at the lower bound of 20 hours. This maximum productivity is approximately 66 % higher than the benchmark experimental study described in Section 6.4 [29]. Moreover, the optimization problem was solved within a total computational solution time of approximately 0.3 seconds. This shows that the model-based optimization approach presented in this chapter is able to predict an improvement in the productivity of recombinant proteins in *P. pastoris*. Therefore, if experiments validate this improvement in productivity, the proposed model-based design

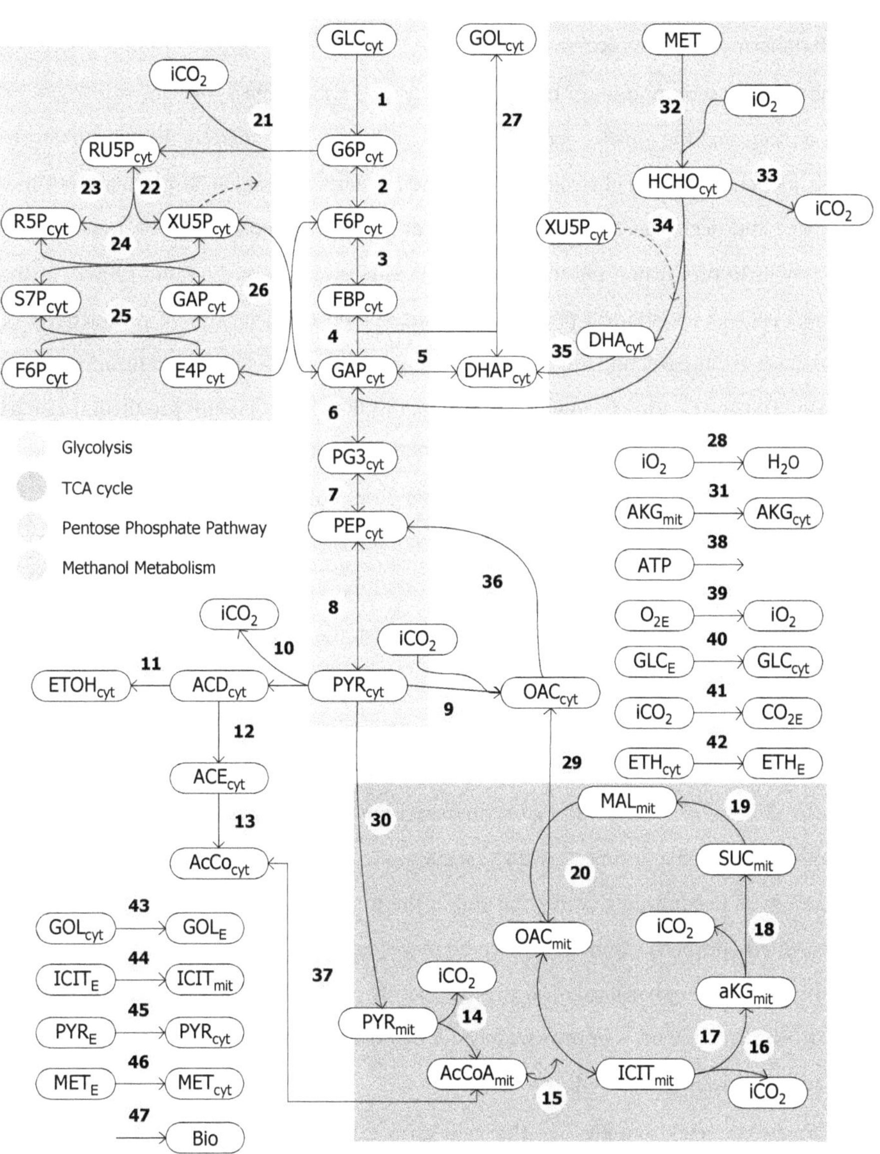

Figure 6.3: Metabolic network of *Pichia pastoris* [49].

framework will reduce the number of costly experiments and facilitate the design of efficient biopharmaceutical processes.

The concentration profiles of the glucose substrate and biomass are shown in Fig. 6.4a. It can be seen that the glucose concentration is gradually consumed by the cells to ensure growth. Concurrently, the glucose substrate feeding starts at a rate of 50 mL/h at the initial time point and decreases slightly to 45 mL/h at t = 18 h to indicate a slow transitioning from growth to production phase (cf. Fig. 6.5). This is to ensure the rapid growth of the *P. pastoris* cells in the shortest possible time, thereby ensuring maximum productivity of recombinant erythropoietin. Rapid cellular growth is crucial for the maximization of the productivity because growth rate is proportional to the erythropoietin production rate as mathematically represented by the Luedeking-Piret model in Section 6.4. From a practical point of view, maximum productivity is favored by rapid cellular growth because recombinant erythropoietin is heterologously expressed and secreted in the host cells [129]. Furthermore, the glucose concentration in the extracellular environment is almost exhausted after 18 hours to indicate the complete transition from the growth phase to the production phase (cf. Fig. 6.4a). Next, a sudden increase in the glucose substrate feeding from 45 to 195 mL/h is observed at the 18-hour mark, maintained at this value for 1 hour before decreasing to approximately zero at the final time $t_f = 20\,\text{h}$ (cf. Fig. 6.5). This sudden increase in glucose feed rate could be to counteract the exhaustion of glucose and cell death in fermentation media at time, $t = 18\,\text{h}$ (see Fig. 6.4a) while ensuring that erythropoietin productivity is maximized towards the end of the process (see Fig. 6.4b). This shows that the presented approach can handle trade-off issues between growth and productivity that typically arise in biopharmaceutical production. It can also be seen on Fig. 6.5 that the highest volume obtained is approximately 1.8 L and therefore within the working volume of 0.5 to 2.0 L stipulated by [29].

It can also be seen from Fig. 6.4a that cells grow exponentially for the first 18 hours and then the biomass concentration decreases slightly towards the end of the fermentation time of 20 hours. This decrease indicates the commencement of proteolytic degradation as described in other studies [30, 119]. Thus, the model-based optimization approach presented in this work is able to predict both the exponential growth and proteolytic degradation that are akin to *P. pastoris* [139, 119].

Moreover, the approach simultaneously predicts all considered intracellular fluxes of *P. pastoris* along with the extracellular fluxes. Fig. 6.6 shows that the intracellular glucose uptake flux follows a similar trend as the extracellular glucose concentration profile (cf. Fig. 6.4a).

Furthermore, the slight decrease in external biomass concentration after 18 hours (Fig. 6.4a) is caused by the intracellular growth rate flux which reaches zero at the same time (Fig. 6.6). On the other hand, the biomass growth rate gradually decreases as the extracellular biomass and substrate concentrations increase and decrease, respectively. However, it can be observed that the biomass concentration increases to 221.27 g/L in 18 hours after which it slightly decreases to 220.20 g/L at the final time. This can be explained by the intracellular growth rate flux which reaches zero at this same time thus implying that cellular growth has stopped (cf. Fig. 6.6).

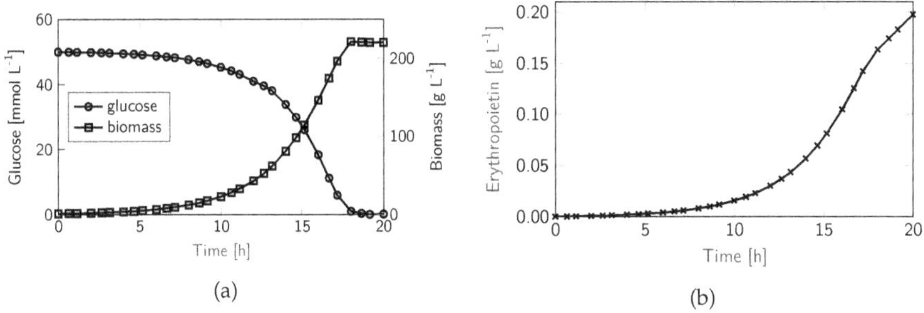

Figure 6.4: Extracellular concentration profiles for the glucose substrate and biomass (a); and the recombinant erythropoietin product (b).

Intracellular fluxes

The optimal dynamic activity of the intracellular fluxes in *P. pastoris* are shown in Fig. 6.7. Details on the metabolic reactions (fluxes) are shown in Fig. 6.3. These dynamic flux distri-

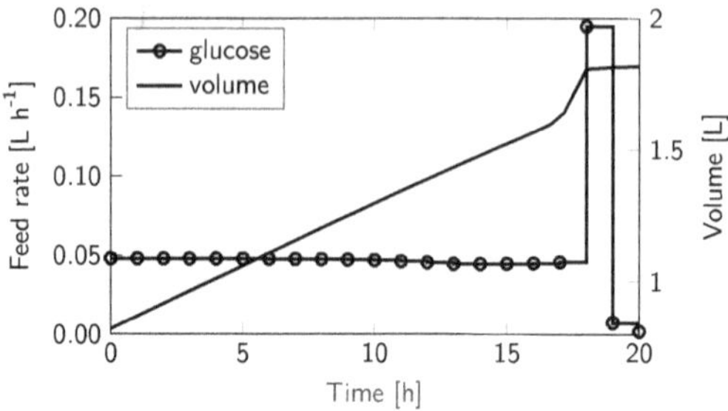

Figure 6.5: Substrate feed rate control and volume profiles.

butions correspond to the optimal metabolic physiological activity required for maximum productivity of erythropoietin.

Note that since methanol and glycerol uptake fluxes are set to zero as described in Section 6.4, fluxes 32 to 35 and 46 corresponding to methanol metabolism and flux 27 corresponding to glycerol formation are inactive throughout the process. In the subsequent sections, the optimal flux evolution of the glycolysis, tricarboxylic acid (TCA) cycle, fermentative, pentose phosphate pathways, and the transport fluxes will be discussed in detail.

Embden–Meyerhoff–Parnas (glycolysis) pathway

First, the flux distributions at the initial time point is considered (cf. Fig. 6.8a). It can be observed that fluxes 1 to 8 corresponding to the Embden Meyerhoff Parnas (EMP) pathway (i.e. glycolysis) are higher at the initial time point $t = 0\,\text{h}$ than at time, $t = 19\,\text{h}$. This implies that for optimal productivity to be achieved, a higher activity of the glycolysis pathway at the onset of the fermentation is required during the exponential growth phase when high cell growth is crucial. This high activity of the EMP pathway plays an important role in the production of energy in the form of ATPs required for the synthesis of organic intermediates and amino acids [188].

Apart from the onset of the fermentation process, the EMP fluxes (fluxes 1 to 8) are active for the majority of the fermentation process until 18 hours where the growth rate

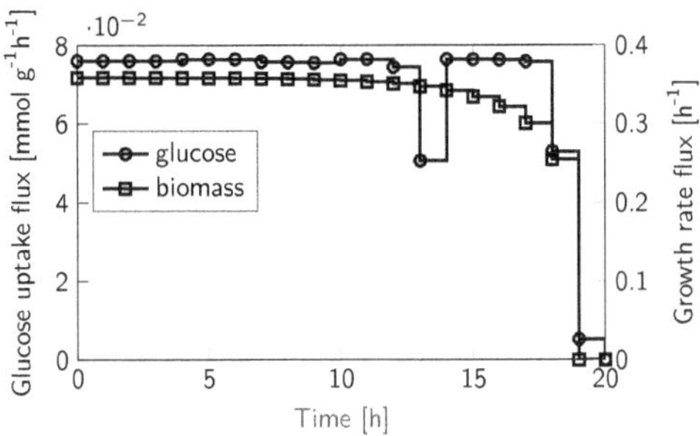

Figure 6.6: Intracellular substrate uptake and growth rate fluxes.

decreases in order to facilitate higher erythropoietin production in the shortest possible time (see Fig. 6.7). On the contrary, towards the end of the process, relatively lower glycolysis fluxes are required for cellular maintenance in order to counteract the cellular burden posed by recombinant protein production [70].

It can also be seen that the fluxes 9 and 10 are inactive for the first 14 hours of the process, but increases slightly towards the end of the process (see Figs. 6.8b and 6.7). Intracellular reactions 9 and 10 correspond to the pathway which drives the formation and consumption of pyruvate, and therefore implies that pyruvate is produced in trace amounts as a by-product at the end of the bioreaction. This validates the claim by other authors that trace amounts of pyruvate are sometimes present in the media when using *P. pastoris* [69, 78]. This implies that for optimal productivity to be ensured, *P. pastoris* strain should be metabolically engineered in such as way that fluxes corresponding to pyruvate formation are inactive. However, more experimental work is required to validate this finding.

Tricarboxylic acid (TCA) cycle

The TCA cycle is an important part of the central carbon metabolism of *P.pastoris* because it produces a majority of the energy required for the synthesis of amino acids used for cell growth [188]. The dynamic intracelluar fluxes in TCA cycle are shown in Fig. 6.7. It can be

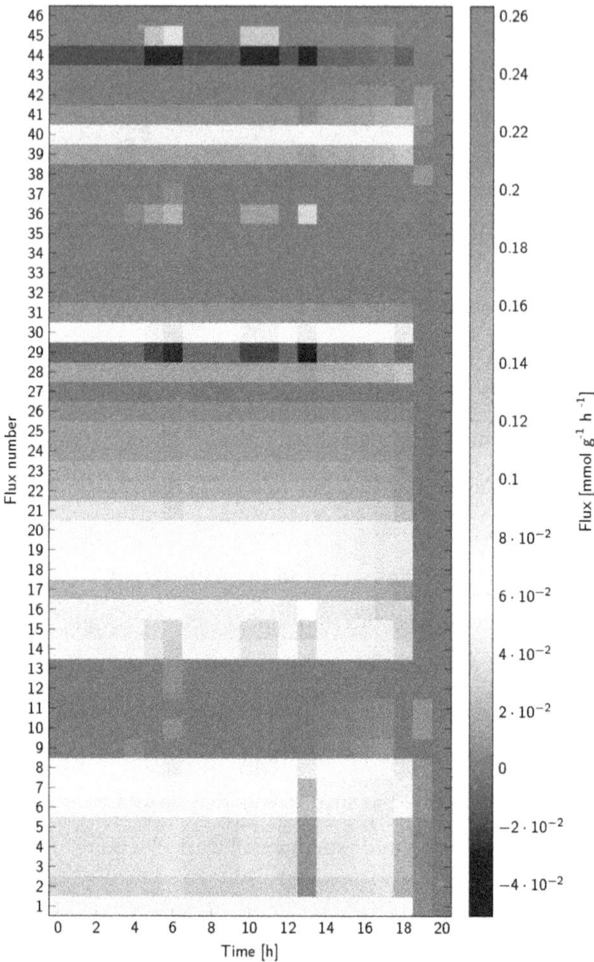

Figure 6.7: Optimal dynamic intracellular fluxes in *P. pastoris*. Flux numbers correspond to the intracellular reactions in Fig. 6.3.

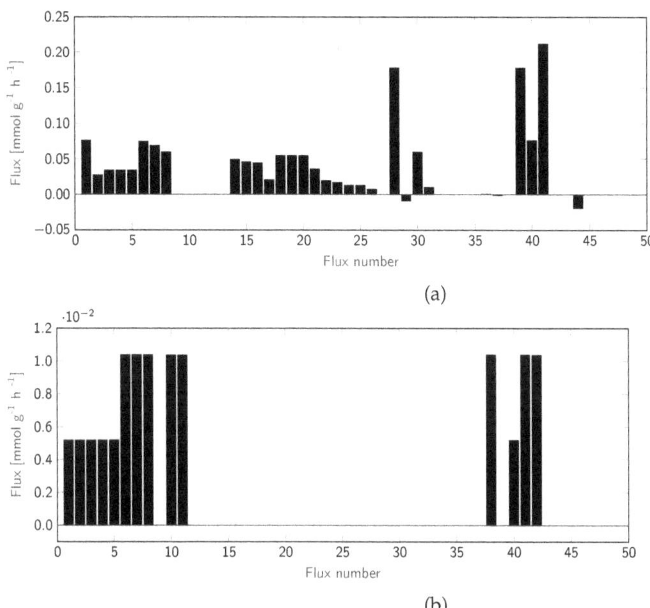

Figure 6.8: Flux distributions at the initial time, $t_0 = 0\,\text{h}$ (a); and at time, $t = 19\,\text{h}$ close to the final time (b). Flux numbers correspond to the intracellular reactions in Fig. 6.3.

Table 6.2: Flux-gene-enzyme mapping (adapted from [122]).

Flux	Gene	Enzyme	Functional category
11	ADH2	Alcohol dehydrogenase	Fermentative pathway
20	MDH1	Malate dehydrogenase	TCA
21	SOL3	6-phosphogluconolactonase	PPP
21	ZWF1	Glucose-6-phosphatedehydrogenase	PPP
22	RPE1	Ribulose-5-phosphate-3- epiremase	PPP
23	RPE1	Ribulose-5-phosphate-3- epiremase	PPP

concluded that the activity of the TCA cycle (fluxes 14 to 20) implies that enough energy is produced during the exponential growth phase, and this energy is simultaneously used to produce amino acids required for cellular growth and recombinant proteins during the production phase (cf. Fig. 6.7).

By looking at Figs. 6.6 and 6.7, it can be seen that the TCA cycle and biomass flux are positively correlated with the exception of time $t = 13\,\text{h}$. Here, it can be observed that the biomass flux decreases while fluxes 18 to 20 increase slightly. This slight increase suggests an increase in energy generation through the TCA cycle for productivity maximization while compensating for low growth rate [70].

As can be noted, the malate dehydrogenase (MDH1) gene (see Table 6.2) which drives flux 20 is active for the most part of the process. [122] state that overexpression and activity of MDH1 might be beneficial for protein production, while [43] suggest that the downregulation or knockout of MDH1 could improve protein synthesis in the fungus *Aspergillus niger*. Due to this discrepancy, [122] have reported that there is no lucid correlation between MDH1 activity and protein production. These results suggest that the activity or inactivity of the MDH1 could depend on the exact time point in the fermentation in which a measurement is taken. Specifically, a dynamic switching between activity and inactivity of the MDH1 gene (flux 20) at the 19-hour mark can be noticed. It might be that the dynamic switching between activity and inactivity of MDH1 could favor optimal erythropoietin production. Furthermore, this could be implemented experimentally by dynamically overexpressing and knocking out the MDH1 gene in the growth and production phases, respectively [25, 26].

Fermentative pathway

The fermentative pathway is represented by fluxes 11 to 13. Fluxes 12 and 13 of the fermentative pathway are inactive throughout time horizon (cf. Fig. 6.7). Flux 11 corresponds to the activity of the alcohol dehydrogenase (ADH2) gene (cf. Table 6.2) which drives the intracellular reaction that results in the production of ethanol in the cytoplasm. Similar to the fluxes 9 and 10 of the pyruvate branch point, flux 11 slightly increases towards the end of the process due to the activity of ADH2; implying that ethanol is formed towards the end of process where cellular burden is high. Since ethanol production could lead to lower erythropoietin productivity, These results suggest that *P. pastoris* can optimally adjust its physiology properly.

This is done in order to ensure that erythropoietin productivity is still maximized towards the end of the process. These results support earlier studies which claim that *P. pastoris* host cells favor the respiratory pathway and as such produce little or no by-products and are less prone to follow the fermentative pathways as in *E. coli* or *S. cerevisiae* [53].

Pentose phosphate pathway (PPP)

The pentose phosphate pathway (PPP) is a part of the central carbon metabolism of *P. pastoris* that utilizes the energy produced from the EMP pathway and TCA cycle to synthesize the amino acids and organic precursors required for biomass synthesis and recombinant protein production. The results for the optimal dynamic intracellular fluxes in PPP (fluxes 21 to 26) are shown in Fig. 6.7.

Here, fluxes 21 to 26 are active throughout the first 18 hours when growth rate is highest (see Figs. 6.6 and 6.7). This is logical as the PPP is a major producer of the amino acids and organic precursors required for biomass synthesis [188]. A close look at Fig. 6.7 reveals that flux 21 which corresponds to the 6-phosphogluconolactonase (SOL3) and glucose-6-phosphatedehydrogenase (ZWF1) genes has the strongest impact on the PPP, and consequently, the biomass and the recombinant erythropoietin protein production. This implies that for maximum productivity, more emphasis should be placed on engineering *P. pastoris* strains such that the activity of the ZWF1 and SOL3 genes are higher than other PPP-associated genes such as ribulose-5-phosphate-3- epiremase (see Table 6.2). Lastly, it can be observed that flux 28 is very high for the first 17 hours but decreases slightly at the 18-hour mark. This is logical because flux 28 represents oxidative phosphorylation which is a reaction that produces energy in the form of ATP that is required for both biomass synthesis and maximum erythropoietin productivity.

Transport fluxes

Transport fluxes (fluxes 29 to 46) facilitate the exchange of metabolites between the *P. pastoris* cell membrane and the extracellular environment, and between the mitochondrion and the cytoplasm within the cell (cf. Fig. 6.7). Flux 31 shows the transport of α-ketoglutarate which serves as an organic precursor for the synthesis of biomass. Even though, flux 31 is very low throughout the process, its presence throughout the growth phase implies that it is still important for maximum biomass synthesis.

Moreover, the cell maintenance is represented by flux 38. It can be seen that there is no need for cellular maintenance during the growth phase. However, as soon as the cell transitions to the production phase at $t = 18\,\mathrm{h}$, the cellular maintenance flux becomes active. This sudden need for cellular maintenance can be attributed to the need for the cell to counteract proteolytic degradation. This is logical and attests to the key insights that can be obtained by using the approach presented in this chapter. It can also be observed that the glucose uptake flux (flux 40) is relatively high until $t = 18\,\mathrm{h}$ (see also Fig. 6.6). Flux 39 which represents the oxygen uptake flux is active and high for the first 18 hours and as a result justifies the assumption that the process is well aerated (see Section 6.4). This implies that for maximum recombinant production, high oxygen rates are required.

Another important finding is the presence of fermentative by-products. Most studies suggest that fermentative by-products such as ethanol, citrate acid or pyruvate are either not produced or produced in little quantities [78, 69]. This is because *P. pastoris* has been known to follow oxidative respiration instead of the fermentative pathway [78, 53]. However, the results in this chapter show that ethanol (flux 42) is excreted to the extracellular environment during the production phase, but not produced during the growth phase (0 to 13 hours). This could be the reason why some authors do not detect ethanol in their studies [171, 31]. Furthermore, the results suggest that citric acid (flux 44) and pyruvate (flux

45) are present during the process. Nonetheless, the presence of fermentative by-products is supported by other studies [70, 69] and NMR experiments [78].

Even though fermentative by-products such as ethanol are considered to be disadvantageous during heterologous protein production, it might be that a little ethanol in the culture media serves as a carbon source when the main carbon sources such as glucose are exhausted, thus improving productivity [194]. This shows that the proposed dFBA approach can provide insights into the underlying biological occurrences in the *P. pastoris* cells; thus, serving as a detailed modeling approach for the design of optimal bioreactors for biopharmaceutical manufacturing.

6.6 SUMMARY

In this chapter, a model-based strategy to optimize the productivity of recombinant protein production by *P. pastoris* has been presented. The external environment is modeled within the EPF framework, while the intracellular metabolic network is modeled with FBA. The approach enables one to gain insights into what dynamic strategies can be implemented at both bioreactor and microorganism scales in order to maximize productivity.

Besides the maximization of productivity, the approach presented herein can be readily extended to other objectives that are of biological relevance. Another key contribution in this work is the efficient solution strategy for the dFBA. It has been shown that dFBA problems can be solved efficiently and directly by replacing the lower-level FBA with its KKT conditions [142], handling the belligerent complementarity constraints with the ℓ_1 penalization technique [9], and solving the dynamic optimization by the simultaneous approach [17].

Therefore, the model-based optimization strategy presented in this chapter is believed to be a valuable contribution to the growing literature on strategies for improving the heterologous expression of proteins in *P. pastoris* and could facilitate the design of next generation biopharmaceutical processes.

7

CONCLUSIONS AND FUTURE DIRECTIONS

This thesis consists of model-based methodologies; based on the concept of elementary process functions (EPF), for the design of optimal reactors for (bio)pharmaceutical manufacturing. The problems considered in this thesis range from the synthesis of APIs and organic intermediates to production of biologics in microorganisms. Moreover, this thesis presents ideas and demonstrates how to adapt the EPF approach for (bio)pharmaceutical manufacturing. By so doing, it has been shown that process systems engineering (PSE) methods are indeed crucial for facilitating Quality by Design. In this concluding chapter, the major contributions and future directions of the research reported in this thesis will be presented.

7.1 CONCLUSIONS

In conclusion, the contributions in this this thesis are summarized below:

Contribution One. Chapter 3 shows for the first time how to adapt the EPF approach to design optimal reactors for the synthesis of APIs and organic intermediates. As a case study, the nucleophilic aromatic substitution of 2,4-difluoronitrobenzene was considered and it was shown that dosing intensification concepts are not beneficial for this case study. Furthermore, key thermodynamic equations such as specific heat capacity equations—

which are required for EPF but usually not available for the complex compounds in API synthesis—were derived by group contribution methods.

Contribution Two. In Chapter 4, the EPF approach was then extended for the first time to the field of enzyme-catalyzed reactions (biocatalysis). As a case study, the enzyme-catalyzed carboligation to produce 2-hydroxy-ketones was considered. On the contrary to results from Chapter 3, it was shown that dosing strategies are beneficial. Moreover, the model-based optimization results by using the EPF concept were validated by experiments; thus demonstrating the viability of the EPF approach for designing optimal reactors for API synthesis via biocatalysis.

Contribution Three. In Chapter 5, the problem of designing robust optimal reactors in the presence of uncertainty was tackled. A novel back-off algorithm for dynamic optimization under parametric uncertainty was presented. This back-off algorithm replaces the Monte Carlo simulations used in determining the statistical moments for calculating the back-offs with the point estimate method (PEM). It was shown that the PEM-based back-off approach is at least 10 times faster than conventional Monte-Carlo based back-off algorithm while maintaining low approximation errors.

Contribution Four. In Chapter 6, a multiscale bioreactor design approach based on dynamic flux balance analysis (dFBA) that was posed within the EPF framework was presented. Here, a novel dFBA solution strategy that combines direct collocation, bilevel optimization reformulation, ℓ_1 penalization, and nonlinear programming was presented. As a case study, the heterologous production of erythropoietin in *Pichia pastoris* was considered. By applying the solution strategy, it was predicted that a 66% increase in productivity could be achieved by an approximately constant feeding profile and the activity the most fluxes in the central carbon metabolism of *P. pastoris*.

7.2 FUTURE RESEARCH DIRECTIONS

Future research One. This thesis lays a foundation on how the EPF approach can be translated to (bio)pharmaceutical applications. Most of the reactors designed in this work fall under the category of established reactors such as plug flow reactors and fed-batch reactors. Even though some reactors designed in this thesis were validated by laboratory experiments; as shown in Chapter 3, it still remains to be seen if the EPF approach can lead to new types of reactors for (bio)pharmaceutical applications.

A possible way forward in this regard will be to use recently proposed flux profile analysis (FPA) [89, 203] to obtain reactor networks for the major classes of reactions used pharmaeutical manufacturing. This can be done in a fast and efficient way and can serve as a look-up table for process engineers in pharmaceutical process development. Based on this look-up table, promising reactor designs for specific reaction classes can then be explored in greater detail by using the EPF method. The FPA approach has been recently proven to lead to novel reactor configurations for chemical production [83, 82]; and therefore has the potential of leading to similar results for (bio)pharmaceutical manufacturing.

Future research Two. There are still some open questions and research opportunities to be pursued based on the results in Chapter 6. For instance, the EPF formulation of the bioreactor design problem presented needs to be explored in greater detail in future studies. A possible direction will be to combine the EPF bioreactor formulation with the three-level reactor design approach proposed by Peschel *et al.* [132]. This could lead to the design of innovative bioreactors that consider the dynamic manipulations of extracellular and intracellular controls for improving the production of biologic drugs in *P. pastoris*.

Another interesting aspect to consider is the oxygen consumption rate. In Chapter 6, it was assumed that sufficient oxygen is available for the cells to grow. Nevertheless, it might be interesting in the future to include an oxygen balance and dissolved oxygen as an additional control variable [62]. In addition, some of the trajectories of the intracellular fluxes are not smooth. Hence, B-splines could be used to parameterize the intracellular fluxes profiles so as to obtain smoothened curves [187].

Future research Three. Most of the intensification strategies considered in this thesis fall in the category of either dosing or heating fluxes. These intensification strategies enable macroscopic control of the process and are thermodynamically inefficient as reported in [128]. Other controls which could lead to precise control of the process at the molecular scale are fluxes such as photo-illumination, microwaves and ultrasound. This could lead to the so called "perfect reactors" [128] and could be interesting to incorporate these fluxes into the EPF framework in future research.

Future research Four. Another possible extension of the work in this thesis is to combine the reactor design methodologies developed in this thesis with separation units to develop optimal process chains for (bio)pharmaceutical manufacturing.

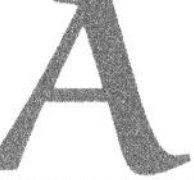

APPENDIX TO CHAPTER 3

A.1 FURTHER RESULTS FOR LEVEL 1

For the second case in the first level (cf. Fig. A.1), reactant **1** starts at a concentration of 0.147 mol/L and reacts instantaneously with **2** at time $t = 0$. As soon as the reaction begins, the remaining portion of **1** is dosed at 0.03 seconds with a molar flow rate of 16.29 mmol/min. This leads to a rapid increase of the concentration of **1** to 0.154 mol/L followed by its gradual decrease along the reaction coordinate as it reacts with **2**. The residence time achieved by using the second concept results in a residence time of 3.22 minutes, and a selectivity of 86 %.

Fig. A.2 shows the results for the third case, the results are quite similar to the results for the second case. However, reactant **2** is dosed instead of **1** in this case. Hence, the initial concentration **2** is 0.442 mol/L but additional moles of **2** are dosed after 0.03 seconds with a molar flow rate of 48.94 mmol/min. The residence time and selectivity are also similar to that obtained in the second case.

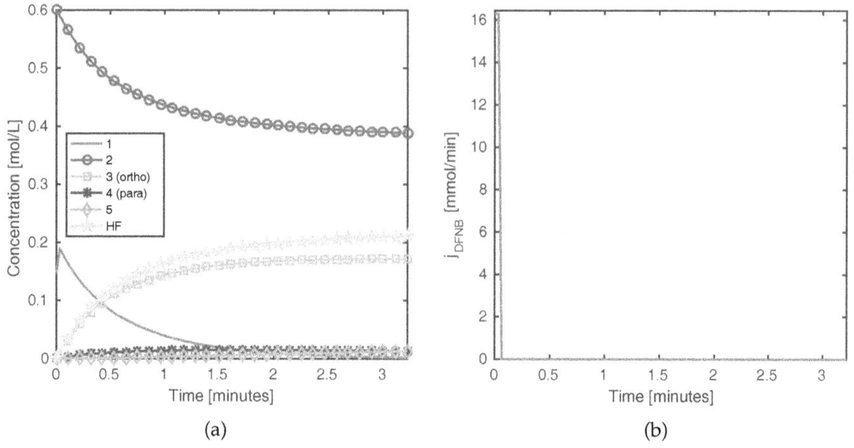

Figure A.1: Optimization results for level 1, case 1 (τ = 3.22 minutes, γ = 3.00): a) concentration state profiles; b) dosing of **1** control profile.

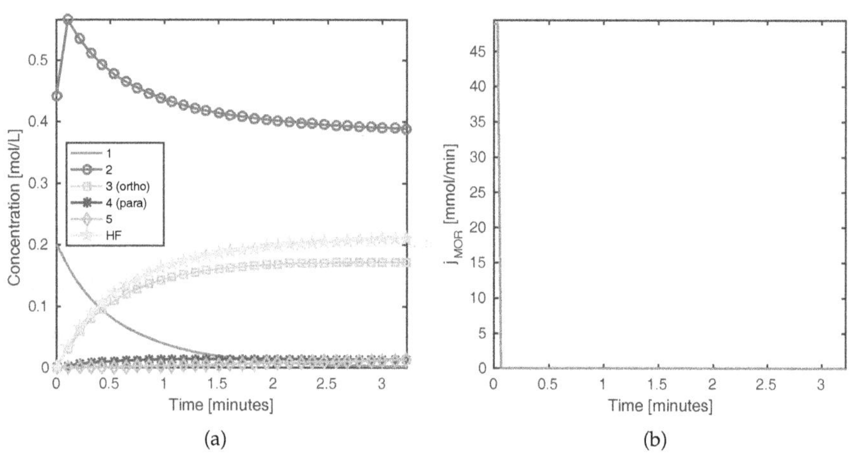

Figure A.2: Optimization results for level 1, case 2 (τ = 3.22 minutes, γ = 3.00): a) concentration state profiles; b) dosing of **2** control profile.

A.2 MODEL ASSUMPTIONS FOR LEVEL 2

The specific heat capacity of the reacting species in Eq. 3.8 are expressed as polynomial functions of temperature. They are obtained by using least squares optimization in cases where experimental data from literature is available and by using group contributions in cases where they are not. Details of how the coefficients of the specific heat capacity equations are obtained are shown in A.3.

The left hand side of the energy balance equation above (cf. Eq. 3.8), is made of contributions from the reacting species and the solvent (ethanol). The energy balance is formulated in such a way that only the specific heat capacities of the reacting species are dependent on temperature while the specific capacity of the solvent is assumed to vary negligibly with temperature. The assumption is valid for two reasons: (1.) the model reaction considered is a homogeneous liquid phase reaction; (2.) a rough *back-of-the-envelope* calculation reveals that the solvent occupies majority of the volume in the reference reactor. Moreover, this assumption reduces complexity of the model and intractable nonlinearities during subsequent optimization. The density of the solvent is also assumed to be constant since the reaction is a homogeneous liquid phase reaction.

A.3 HEAT CAPACITY

In this work, two approaches were used to obtain the specific heat capacity c_p equations. In the first approach, when specific heat capacity data are available in literature for a compound i, it is assumed that $c_{p,i}(T)$ follows a polynomial function of degree 2 as it provides a compromise between data fitting (see Fig. A.3 and A.4) and numerical robustness, i.e. avoiding overfitting and Runge's phenomenon:

$$c_{p,i}(T) = \alpha_i + \beta_i T + \gamma_i T^2. \tag{A.1}$$

Based on this polynomial function, least squares optimization [22] is performed to estimate the coefficients α_i, β_i, and γ_i

$$\min \ \|\mathbf{A}_i\hat{\mathbf{x}}_i - \mathbf{b}_i\|^2 \tag{A.2}$$

where

$\mathbf{A}_i\hat{\mathbf{x}}_i - \mathbf{b}_i$ is the residual or error,

$\mathbf{b}_i = (c_{p,i,1}, c_{p,i,2}, ..., c_{p,i,k})$ is the specific heat capacities (outcomes) measured at different temperatures (observables) k,

$\hat{\mathbf{x}}_i = (\alpha_i, \beta_i, \gamma_i) \in \mathbb{R}^3$ is a vector containing the least-squares estimated coefficients for component i and

$\mathbf{A}_i \in \mathbb{R}^{k\times 3}$ is a Vandermonde matrix with ($k \geq 3$).

$$\mathbf{A} = \begin{bmatrix} 1 & T_1 & T_1^2 \\ 1 & T_2 & T_2^2 \\ \vdots & \vdots & \vdots \\ 1 & T_k & T_k^2 \end{bmatrix} \tag{A.3}$$

The first approach was used to obtain the specific heat capacity equations for morpholine (2) [114] and hydrogen fluoride (HF) [76] (see Fig. A.4 and A.3).

For the other components for which specific heat capacity data could not be found, a group contribution method [147] given by the following equation was used:

$$c_{p,i}(T) = \sum_i n_i a_i + \sum_i n_i b_i T + \sum_i n_i c_i T^2 + \sum_i n_i d_i T^3 \tag{A.4}$$

where n_i is the number of occurrence of group i in a given molecule, a_i, b_i, c_i, and d_i are semi-empirical values associated with the group i, and T is the absolute temperature. Based on these two approaches, the coefficients for the specific heat equation for each compound are given in Table A.1.

Table A.1: Coefficients of specific heat capacity equations [100].

Species	α [J/(mol K)]	β [J/(mol K^2)]	γ [J/(mol K^3)]	δ [J/mol K^4]
1†	-1.912×10^1	5.700×10^{-1}	-3.761×10^{-4}	8.787×10^{-8}
2‡	-1.712×10^{-3}	8.447×10^0	-1.198×10^{-2}	–
3†	-6.654×10^1	1.075×10^0	-7.132×10^{-4}	1.660×10^{-7}
4†	-6.654×10^1	1.075×10^0	-7.132×10^{-4}	1.660×10^{-7}
5†	-1.139×10^2	1.579×10^0	-1.050×10^{-3}	2.441×10^{-7}
HF‡	6.251×10^1	-2.229×10^{-1}	6.294×10^{-4}	–
EtOH$^\diamondsuit$	1.124×10^3	–	–	–

† coefficients obtained from group contribution methods. ‡ coefficients obtained from least-squares optimization. ◇ a constant value was used.

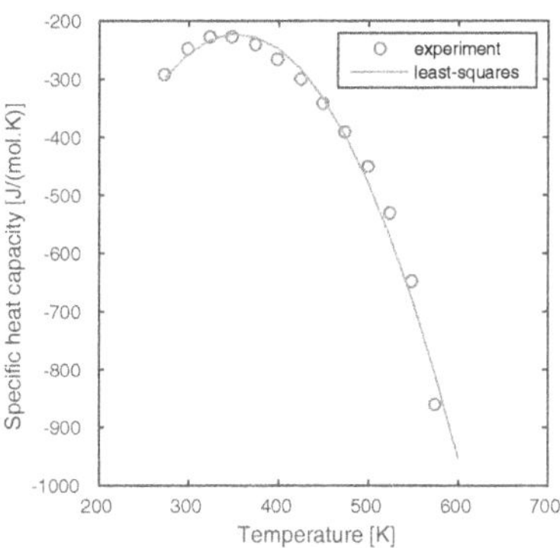

Figure A.3: Determining the coefficients of the specific heat capacity equation for morpholine. The coefficients were determined by applying a second-order least square approximation on the experimental data from Mesmer and Hitch [114]. is that for the ionization of morpholine at saturation pressure of water at infinite dilution.

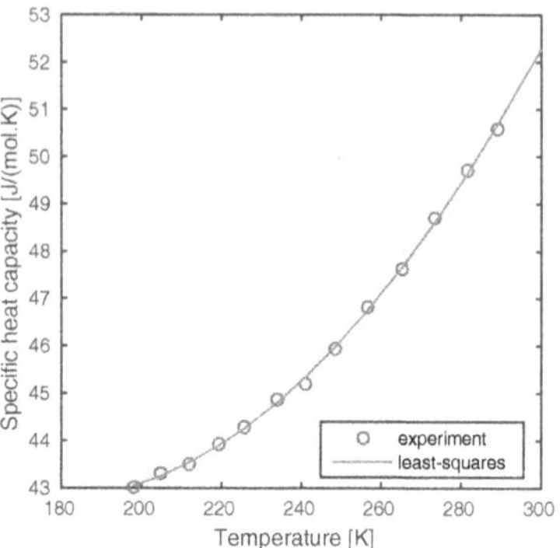

Figure A.4: Determining the coefficients of the specific heat capacity equation for hydrogen fluoride. These coefficients were determined by applying a second-order least square approximation on experimental data [76].

A.4 DETAILED MODEL DEVELOPMENT FOR LEVEL 3

A detailed derivation of the coolant temperature T_e in level 3 reads as:

$$\frac{A_e \cdot v_e \cdot \rho_e \cdot c_{p,e}}{\mathrm{Mwt_e}} \frac{dT_e}{dz} = \frac{\pi d_e}{A_e} \cdot j_q \tag{A.5}$$

K_e is an aggregated cooling fluid-dependent parameter that ranges from -1 to 1 min dm K/J [132, 133] and it is given as:

$$K_e = \frac{\pi \cdot d_e \cdot \mathrm{Mwt_e}}{A_e \cdot v_e \cdot \rho_e \cdot c_{p,e}} \tag{A.6}$$

where $\mathrm{Mwt_e}$ is the molecular weight of the (cooling or heating) environment fluid, d_e is the diameter of the tube around the reactor in which the environment fluid flows, A_e is the is the cross-sectional area of the jacket around the reactor, v_e is the velocity of the environment fluid, ρ_e is the density of the environment fluid, and $c_{p,e}$ is the specific heat capacity of the environment fluid. These aforementioned parameters are assumed to be constant.

The solvent is also assumed to occupy a significant portion of the volume of the reactor. Based on this assumption, it suffices to assume that the Reynolds number will largely depend on the flow of the solvent (ethanol, EtOH).

B

APPENDIX TO CHAPTER 5

B.1 RESULTS FOR THE REFERENCE CASE: BATCH REACTOR

The concentration profiles of the batch reactor are shown in Fig. B.1. For this case, the final concentration of the target product BA is 3.11 $\mathrm{mmol\,L^{-1}}$ (see Table 5.2). Here, propanal (A) starts at a concentration of 11.16 $\mathrm{mmol\,L^{-1}}$ and then decreases gradually to 8.05 $\mathrm{mmol\,L^{-1}}$. Concurrently, benzaldehyde (B) starts at 6.61 $\mathrm{mmol\,L^{-1}}$ and decreases at a faster rate in comparison to reactant A to 0.55 $\mathrm{mmol\,L^{-1}}$. It can be seen that the optimal initial concentration of A is higher than that of B. This is logical as the rate equations and molar balances reveal a proportional relationship between reactant A and the target product BA. First, every consumption of A leads to a formation of AB. Therefore, a high A concentration maximizes AB. As B may also form BB, its rate is faster than for A. However, to minimize losses to BB, a lower concentration of B is chosen. This can also be seen in the reaction scheme 4.1 and in the rate equations.

Furthermore, the enzyme concentration starts at the upper bound of 50 $\mathrm{\mu g^{-1}mL}$ for similar reasons as in Section 5.4. Another key observation is that the concentration of BA is almost maximized after the enzyme inactivates. This is due to two reasons. First, the benzaldehyde self-carboligation step appears to have reached an equilibrium, and the inactivity of the enzyme implies that the cross-carboligation reaction to produce BA is inhibited.

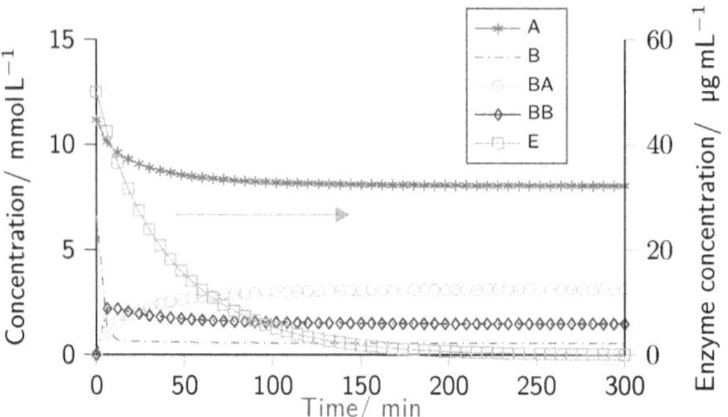

Figure B.1: Nominal dynamic optimization results for the reference batch reactor case: concentration profiles.

B.2 RESULTS FOR CASE 1: DOSING OF PROPANAL

With the results of the batch case delineated, the effect of dosing only propanal (A) along the reaction route will now be discussed (see Fig. B.2). By dosing A, the final concentration of (*R*)-2-hydroxy-1-phenylbutan-1-one (BA) achieved is 3.18 mmol L^{-1} (cf. Table 5.2). This is a marginal improvement of 2.25 % over the reference batch case. In Fig. B.2, a non-intuitive concentration profile in comparison to the results of the batch reactor reference case is observed. Here, reactant A starts at a concentration of 3.65 mmol L^{-1} which is lower than the initial concentration of B in this case. The initial concentration of B is 6.51 mmol L^{-1} which is very similar to that of the reference case.

However, it can be noticed that concentration of A decreases to 2.96 mmol L^{-1} after 6 minutes at which point the product BB is maximized. Afterward, the dosing of A is initiated, thus leading to an increase in the concentration of reactant A during the reaction. This is a non-intuitive strategy that requires some more explanation. First, reactant A has to be started at a lower concentration in this case because the optimizer recognized that dosing would be required after 6 minutes to maximize the formation of BA. However, starting A at a higher concentration similar to that of reference case might lead to faster inactivation of the enzyme and thus a lower final product. As a result, the optimizer detects 3.65 $mmol\,L^{-1}$ as the optimal initial concentration for B.

With regards to the decrease in A in the first 6 minutes, it can be observed that this increase coincides with the maximum concentration of the side product BB (at 2.36 $mmol\,L^{-1}$). Afterward, BB starts to decrease due to a reverse reaction as illustrated in Fig. 4.1. This leads to a "domino effect" in which the reverse reaction to produce B is triggered to ensure that sufficient B is maintained in the reaction medium to react with A to produce BA.

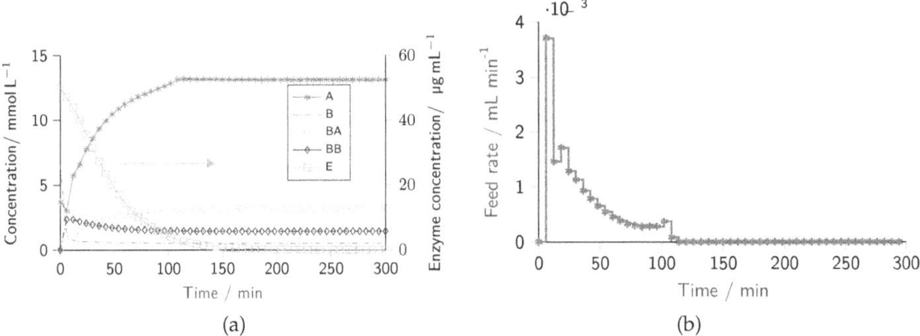

Figure B.2: Nominal dynamic optimization results for the intensification Case 1 involving the dosing of propanal (A). Concentration profiles (states) (a); Feed rate of A as a control (b).

Consequently, the concentration of A is increased by dosing A so that it can continuously react with the almost constant concentration of B to produce as much BA as fast as possible. Similar to the reference case, it can be noticed that the reaction between A and B is halted and that the concentration of BA reaches a constant value as soon as the enzyme is inactivated. For similar reasons, the inactivation of the enzyme implies that the reaction between A and B can no longer be catalyzed and thus, the formation of BA stops. Furthermore, the dosing of A stops at the same time the enzyme is inactivated. This is rational as there is no need to keep feeding propanal if the enzyme is not active to catalyze its reaction with benzaldehyde. Unfortunately, dosing A adversely affects the enzyme activity, i.e., the enzyme inactivates after approximately 138 minutes of reaction which is shorter than the time (about 180 minutes) it takes for the enzyme to inactivate for the reference case. Overall, the final concentration of BA is slightly improved by dosing propanal.

B.3 RESULTS FOR CASE 2: DOSING OF BENZALDEHYDE

As seen in Fig. B.3a, the case of dosing only benzaldehyde (B) yields similar concentration profiles like the reference case. The optimal initial concentrations of A and B are 11.94 and 1.92 mmol L^{-1}, respectively. By dosing only B, the final BA concentration of 3.52 mmol L^{-1} is achieved (cf. Table 5.2). This results in a 13.18 % increase over the reference case. It can be seen that it is more advantageous to dose B in comparison to A. The reason for this increase in comparison to the reference case and the case in which only A was dosed is primarily due to the optimal selection of the initial concentration and the dosing trajectories of B.

In this case, the optimal initial concentration of B is approximately three times lower than those in the batch reference and the intensification Case 1, i.e., dosing of propanal. Here, the rate at which BB is formed is kept lower than the two previous cases by ensuring that a lower amount of B is allowed to bind to the enzyme. Despite this lower concentration, an appropriate amount of B which ultimately leads to the maximization of $C_{BA}(t_f)$ is ensured by an optimal feed rate that starts high and gradually decreases along the reaction coordinate (cf. Fig. B.3b). Furthermore, the lower amount of B present during the reaction ensures that the rate of enzyme inactivation due to B is slower. Consequently, the presence of a slightly higher concentration of the enzyme during the reaction leads to the higher concentration of BA.

B.4 TIME-VARYING FORWARD PROPAGATION OF UNCERTAINTY WITH THE NOMINAL CONTROL

In this section, spaghetti plots showing the full propagation of uncertainty with time for all the concentration states (C_A, C_B,C_{BA}, C_{BB} and C_E) considered in Chapter 5 are presented.

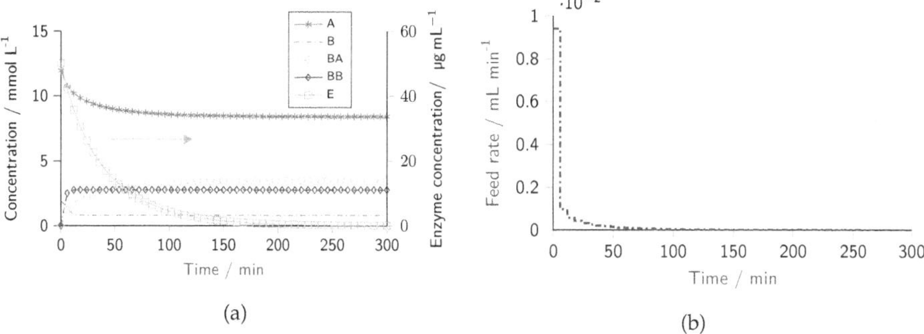

Figure B.3: Nominal dynamic optimization results for the intensification Case 2 involving the dosing of benzaldehyde (B). Concentration profiles (states) (a); Feed rate of B as a control (b).

As already explained these plots were generated by running 2000 Monte Carlo samples. Fig. B.4 shows that upper bound of the benzoin concentration (C_{BB}) was violated, while all the concentration of all other species were well within their respective bounds—for the Monte Carlo scenarios considered.

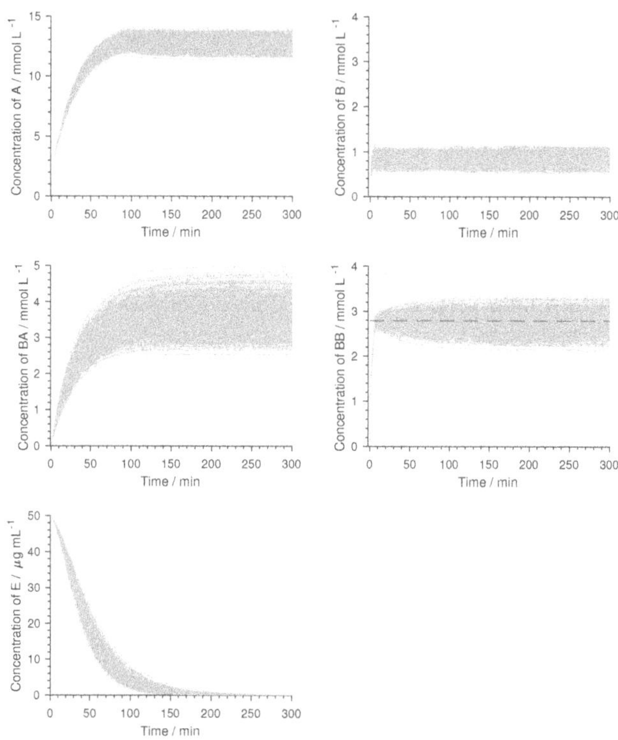

Figure B.4: Concentrations for 2000 forward Monte Carlo simulations using the nominal control profiles for the case of dosing A and B (i.e. case 3). The dotted red line is the upper bound (solubility limit) for BB, and the grey lines the 2000 Monte Carlo simulations. Please note, that the upper bounds for A, B, BA and E are not shown as they are all well within their respective upper bounds.

B.5 SPARSITY PATTERNS

Here, the sparsity patterns of the Jacobian and Hessian matrices for the *Pf*BAL-catalyzed EPF dynamic optimization problem are shown in Fig. B.5. These matrices are very sparse because the dynamic optimization problem depends on relatively small subset of its variables. As mentioned in Section 5.3, the sparsity and structure of Jacobian and Hessian matrices are exploited by the IPOPT algorithm in order to solve the NLP problems faster.

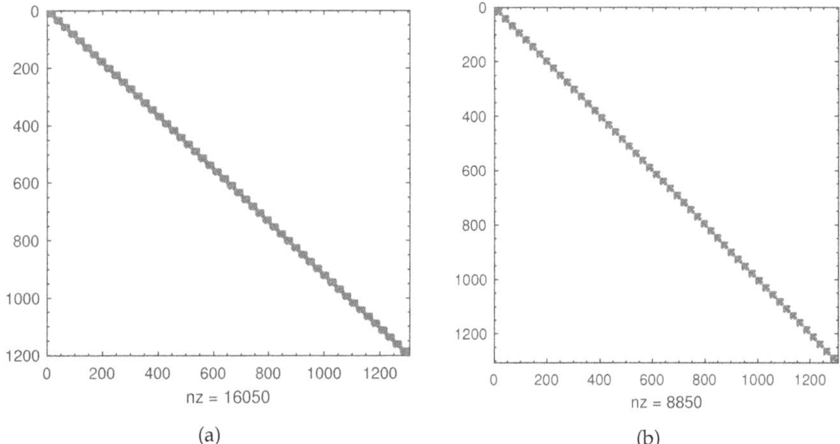

Figure B.5: Karush-Kuhn-Tucker (KKT) sparsity patterns for discretized NLP for the *Pf*BAL-catalyzed EPF formulation, where nz means the number of non-zeros. Jacobian matrix (a); Hessian matrix (b).

BIBLIOGRAPHY

[1] L. Achenie and L. T. Biegler. A superstructure based approach to chemical reactor network synthesis. *Computers & Chemical Engineering*, 14(1):23–40, 1990. URL http://dx.doi.org/10.1016/0098-1354(90)87003-8.

[2] S. R. Aggarwal. What's fueling the biotech engine–2012 to 2013. *Nature*, 32(1):32–39, 2014. URL http://dx.doi.org/10.1038/nbt.2794.

[3] J. A. E. Andersson, J. Gillis, G. Horn, J. B. Rawlings, and M. Diehl. CasADi: a software framework for nonlinear optimization and optimal control. *Mathematical Programming Computation*, 2018. URL http://link.springer.com/10.1007/s12532-018-0139-4.

[4] N. Anesiadis, W. R. Cluett, and R. Mahadevan. Dynamic metabolic engineering for increasing bioprocess productivity. *Metabolic Engineering*, 10(5):255–266, 2008. URL https://doi.org/10.1016/j.ymben.2008.06.004.

[5] F. H. Arnold. Directed evolution: Bringing new chemistry to life. *Angewandte Chemie International Edition*, pages 2–8, 2017. URL http://doi.wiley.com/10.1002/anie.201708408.

[6] E. Aydin, D. Bonvin, and K. Sundmacher. NMPC using Pontryagin's Minimum Principle-Application to a two-phase semi-batch hydroformylation reactor under uncertainty. *Computers & Chemical Engineering*, 108:47–56, 2018. URL http://dx.doi.org/10.1016/j.compchemeng.2017.08.010.

[7] R. A. Bakker and H. E. A. Van den Akker. A lagrangian description of micromixing in a stirred tank reactor using 1d-micromixing model in a CFD flow field. *Chemical engineering science*, 51(11):2643–2648, 1996. URL http://dx.doi.org/10.1016/0009-2509(96)00130-3.

[8] P. Barthe, C. Guermeur, O. Lobet, M. Moreno, P. Woehl, D. M. Roberge, N. Bieler, and B. Zimmermann. Continuous multi-injection reactor for multipurpose production–part I. *Chemical Engineering & Technology*, 31(8):1146–1154, 2008. URL http://dx.doi.org/10.1002/ceat.200800132.

[9] B. T. Baumrucker, J. G. Renfro, and L. T. Biegler. MPEC problem formulations and solution strategies with chemical engineering applications. *Computers & Chemical Engineering*, 32(12):2903–2913, 2008. URL http://dx.doi.org/10.1016/j.compchemeng.2008.02.010.

[10] I. R. Baxendale. The integration of flow reactors into synthetic organic chemistry. *Journal of Chemical Technology and Biotechnology*, 88(4):519–552, 2013. URL http://dx.doi.org/10.1002/jctb.4012.

[11] J. Begemann, R. B. Ohs, A. B. Ogolong, W. Eberhard, M. B. Ansorge-Schumacher, and A. C. Spiess. Model-based analysis of a reactor and control concept for oxidoreductions based on exhaust CO_2-measurement. *Process Biochemistry*, 51(10):1397–1405, 2016. URL http://dx.doi.org/10.1016/j.procbio.2016.06.024.

[12] R. Bellman. On the theory of dynamic programming. *Proceedings of the National Academy of Sciences*, 38(8):716–719, 1952.

[13] L. Bergner and C. Kirches. The polynomial chaos approach for reachable set propagation with application to chance-constrained nonlinear optimal control under parametric uncertainties. *Optimal Control Applications and Methods*, 39(2):471–488, 2018. URL http://doi.wiley.com/10.1002/oca.2329.

[14] D. P. Bertsekas and J. N. Tsitsiklis. *Introduction to Probability*. Athena Scientific, 2 edition, 2008. ISBN 978-1-886529-23-6.

[15] L. T. Biegler. Solution of dynamic optimization problems by successive quadratic programming and orthogonal collocation. *Computers & Chemical Engineering*, 8(3-4): 243–247, 1984. URL https://doi.org/10.1016/0098-1354(84)87012-X.

[16] L. T. Biegler. Solution of dynamic optimization problems by successive quadratic programming and orthogonal collocation. *Computers & Chemical Engineering*, 8(3-4): 243–247, 1984. URL https://doi.org/10.1016/0098-1354(84)87012-X.

[17] L. T. Biegler. An overview of simultaneous strategies for dynamic optimization. *Chemical Engineering and Processing: Process Intensification*, 46(11):1043–1053, 2007. URL https://doi.org/10.1016/j.cep.2006.06.021.

[18] L. T. Biegler. *Nonlinear Programming*. Society for Industrial and Applied Mathematics, Philadelphia, 2010. ISBN 978-0-89871-702-0. URL http://epubs.siam.org/doi/book/10.1137/1.9780898719383.

[19] H. G. Bock and K.-J. Plitt. A multiple shooting algorithm for direct solution of optimal control problems. *IFAC Proceedings Volumes*, 17(2):1603–1608, 1984. URL http://dx.doi.org/10.1016/S1474-6670(17)61205-9.

[20] A. R. Bogdan, S. L. Poe, D. C. Kubis, S. J. Broadwater, and D. T. McQuade. The continuous-flow synthesis of ibuprofen. *Angewandte Chemie International Edition*, 48 (45):8547–8550, 2009. URL http://doi.wiley.com/10.1002/anie.200903055.

[21] B. A. Boghigian, G. Seth, R. Kiss, and B. A. Pfeifer. Metabolic flux analysis and pharmaceutical production. *Metabolic Engineering*, 12(2):81–95, 2010. URL http://dx.doi.org/10.1016/j.ymben.2009.10.004.

[22] S. Boyd and L. Vandenberghe. *Convex Optimization*. Cambridge University Press, New York, 2004.

[23] S. Boyd and L. Vandenberghe. *Introduction to Applied Linear Algebra: Vectors, Matrices, and Least Squares*. Cambridge University Press, 2018. ISBN 9781316518960.

[24] M. Braun, H. Link, L. Liu, R. D. Schmid, and D. Weuster-Botz. Biocatalytic process optimization based on mechanistic modeling of cholic acid oxidation with cofactor regeneration. *Biotechnology and Bioengineering*, 108(6):1307–1317, 2011. URL http://doi.wiley.com/10.1002/bit.23047.

[25] I. M. Brockman and K. L. Prather. Dynamic knockdown of *E. coli* central metabolism for redirecting fluxes of primary metabolites. *Metabolic Engineering*, 28:104–113, 2015. URL http://doi.org/10.1016/j.ymben.2014.12.005.

[26] I. M. Brockman and K. L. J. Prather. Dynamic metabolic engineering: New strategies for developing responsive cell factories. *Biotechnology Journal*, 10(9):1360–1369, 2015. URL http://doi.org/10.1016/10.1002/biot.201400422.

[27] D. L. Browne, B. J. Deadman, R. Ashe, I. R. Baxendale, and S. V. Ley. Continuous flow processing of slurries: evaluation of an agitated cell reactor. *Organic Process Research & Development*, 15(3):693–697, 2011. URL http://dx.doi.org/10.1021/op2000223.

[28] P. Çalık, M. Şahin, H. Taşpınar, E. Ş. Soyaslan, and B. İnankur. Dynamic flux balance analysis for pharmaceutical protein production by *Pichia pastoris*: Human growth hormone. *Enzyme and Microbial Technology*, 48(3):209–216, 2011. URL http://dx.doi.org/10.1016/j.enzmictec.2010.09.016.

[29] E. Çelik, P. Çalık, and S. G. Oliver. Fed-batch methanol feeding strategy for recombinant protein production by *Pichia pastoris* in the presence of co-substrate sorbitol. *Yeast*, 26(9):473–484, 2009. URL http://dx.doi.org/10.1002/yea.1679.

[30] E. Çelik, P. Çalık, and S. G. Oliver. A structured kinetic model for recombinant protein production by Mut+ strain of *Pichia pastoris*. *Chemical Engineering Science*, 64(23):5028–5035, 2009.

[31] E. Çelik, P. Çalık, and S. G. Oliver. Metabolic flux analysis for recombinant protein production by *Pichia pastoris* using dual carbon sources: Effects of methanol feeding rate. *Biotechnology and Bioengineering*, 105(2):317–329, 2010. URL http://dx.doi.org/10.1002/bit.22543.

[32] G. P. L. Cereghino, J. L. Cereghino, C. Ilgen, and J. M. Cregg. Production of recombinant proteins in fermenter cultures of the yeast *Pichia pastoris*. *Current Opinion in Biotechnology*, 13(4):329–332, 2002. URL http://dx.doi.org/10.1016/S0958-1669(02)00330-0.

[33] J. L. Cereghino and J. M. Cregg. Heterologous protein expression in the methylotrophic yeast *Pichia pastoris*. *FEMS Microbiology Reviews*, 24(1):45–66, 2000. URL https://doi.org/10.1111/j.1574-6976.2000.tb00532.x.

[34] M. Charaschanya, A. R. Bogdan, Y. Wang, and S. W. Djuric. Nucleophilic aromatic substitution of heterocycles using a high-temperature and high-pressure flow reactor. *Tetrahedron Letters*, 57(9):1035–1039, 2016. URL http://dx.doi.org/10.1016/j.tetlet.2016.01.080.

[35] B. Chen, S. Lim, A. Kannan, S. C. Alford, F. Sunden, D. Herschlag, I. K. Dimov, T. M. Baer, and J. R. Cochran. High-throughput analysis and protein engineering using microcapillary arrays. *Nature Chemical Biology*, 12(2):76–81, 2016. URL http://dx.doi.org/10.1038/nchembio.1978.

[36] K. M. Christensen, M. J. Pedersen, K. Dam-Johansen, T. L. Holm, T. Skovby, and S. Kiil. Design and operation of a filter reactor for continuous production of a selected pharmaceutical intermediate. *Chemical Engineering Science*, 71:111–117, 2012. URL http://dx.doi.org/10.1016/j.ces.2011.12.002.

[37] P. C. Collins. Chemical engineering and the culmination of quality by design in pharmaceuticals. *AIChE Journal*, 64(5):1502–1510, 2018. URL http://dx.doi.org/10.1002/aic.16154.

[38] B. Colson, P. Marcotte, and G. Savard. An overview of bilevel optimization. *Annals of Operations Research*, 153(1):235–256, 2007. URL http://dx.doi.org/10.1007/s10479-007-0176-2.

[39] O. Cos, R. Ramon, J. L. Montesinos, and F. Valero. A simple model-based control for *Pichia pastoris* allows a more efficient heterologous protein production bioprocess. *Biotechnology and Bioengineering*, 95(1):145–154, 2006. URL http://dx.doi.org/10.1002/bit.21005.

[40] J. E. Cuthrell and L. T. Biegler. On the optimization of differential-algebraic process systems. *AIChE Journal*, 33(8):1257–1270, 1987. URL http://doi.wiley.com/10.1002/aic.690330804.

[41] M. C. d'Anjou and A. J. Daugulis. A rational approach to improving productivity in recombinant *Pichia pastoris* fermentation. *Biotechnology and Bioengineering*, 72(1):1–11, 2001. URL http://dx.doi.org/10.1002/1097-0290(20010105)72:1<1::AID-BIT1>3.0.CO;2-T.

[42] M. Diehl, H. G. Bock, and E. Kostina. An approximation technique for robust nonlinear optimization. *Mathematical Programming*, 107(1-2):213–230, 2006. URL http://link.springer.com/10.1007/s10107-005-0685-1.

[43] H. Driouch, G. Melzer, and C. Wittmann. Integration of *in vivo* and *in silico* metabolic fluxes for improvement of recombinant protein production. *Metabolic Engineering*, 14 (1):47–58, 2012. URL https://doi.org/10.1016/j.ymben.2011.11.002.

[44] A. S. Drud. CONOPT–a large-scale GRG code. *ORSA Journal on computing*, 6(2): 207–216, 1994. URL http://dx.doi.org/10.1287/ijoc.6.2.207.

[45] I. S. Duff. MA57—a code for the solution of sparse symmetric definite and indefinite systems. *ACM Transactions on Mathematical Software*, 30(2):118–144, 2004. URL http://dx.doi.org/10.1145/992200.992202.

[46] A. El Sibai, L. K. Rihko Struckmann, and K. Sundmacher. Model-based optimal sabatier reactor design for power-to-gas applications. *Energy Technology*, 5(6):911–921, 2017. URL http://doi.wiley.com/10.1002/ente.201600600.

[47] V. N. Emenike and U. Krewer. Model-based optimal design of continuous-flow reactors for the synthesis of active pharmaceutical ingredients. *Chemie Ingenieur Technik*, 88(9):1215–1216, 2016. URL https://dx.doi.org/10.1002/cite.201650267.

[48] V. N. Emenike, R. Schenkendorf, and U. Krewer. Model-based optimization of the recombinant protein production in *Pichia pastoris* based on dynamic flux balance analysis and elementary process functions. In M. G. Antonio Espuña and L. Puigjaner, editors, *27th European Symposium on Computer Aided Process Engineering*, Computer Aided Chemical Engineering, pages 2815–2820. Elsevier, 2017. URL https://dx.doi.org/10.1016/B978-0-444-63965-3.50471-2.

[49] V. N. Emenike, R. Schenkendorf, and U. Krewer. Model-based optimization of biopharmaceutical manufacturing in *Pichia pastoris* based on dynamic flux balance analysis. *Computers & Chemical Engineering*, 118:1–13, 2018. URL https://doi.org/10.1016/j.compchemeng.2018.07.013.

[50] V. N. Emenike, R. Schenkendorf, and U. Krewer. A systematic reactor design approach for the synthesis of active pharmaceutical ingredients. *European Journal of Pharmaceutics and Biopharmaceutics*, 126:75–88, 2018. URL https://doi.org/10.1016/j.ejpb.2017.05.007.

[51] V. N. Emenike, D. Hertwig, R. Ohs, R. Schenkendorf, A. C. Spiess, and U. Krewer. A rigorous model-driven approach for the optimal design of reaction strategies for enzyme catalysis. In Preparation, 2019.

[52] V. N. Emenike, X. Xie, R. Schenkendorf, A. C. Spiess, and U. Krewer. Robust dynamic optimization of enzyme-catalyzed carboligation: a point estimate-based back-off approach. *Computers & Chemical Engineering*, 121:232–247, 2019.

[53] M. L. Fazenda, J. M. Dias, L. M. Harvey, A. Nordon, R. Edrada-Ebel, D. LittleJohn, and B. McNeil. Towards better understanding of an industrial cell factory: investigating the feasibility of real-time metabolic flux analysis in *Pichia pastoris*. *Microbial Cell Factories*, 12:51, 2013. URL http://doi.org/10.1186/1475-2859-12-51.

[54] H. S. Fogler. *Elements of chemical reaction engineering*. Prentice-Hall, 4th edition edition, 2006.

[55] R. Fourer, D. Gay, and B. Kernighan. *AMPL. A Modelling Language for Mathematical Programming*. Brooks/Cole Publishing Company, 2nd edition edition, 2003.

[56] H. Freund and K. Sundmacher. Towards a methodology for the systematic analysis and design of efficient chemical processes. *Chemical Engineering and Processing: Process Intensification*, 47(12):2051–2060, 2008. URL https://doi.org/10.1016/j.cep.2008.07.011.

[57] F. Galvanin, M. Barolo, F. Bezzo, and S. Macchietto. A backoff strategy for model-based experiment design under parametric uncertainty. *AIChE Journal*, 56(8):2088–2102, 2009. URL http://doi.wiley.com/10.1002/aic.12138.

[58] H. P. L. Gemoets, Y. Su, M. Shang, V. Hessel, R. Luque, and T. Noël. Liquid phase oxidation chemistry in continuous-flow microreactors. *Chemical Society Reviews*, 45 (1):83–117, 2016. URL http://dx.doi.org/10.1039/C5CS00447K.

[59] K. V. Gernaey, A. E. Cervera-Padrell, and J. M. Woodley. A perspective on PSE in pharmaceutical process development and innovation. *Computers & Chemical Engineering*, 42:15–29, 2012. URL http://dx.doi.org/10.1016/j.compchemeng.2012.02.022.

[60] D. I. Gerogiorgis and H. G. Jolliffe. Continuous pharmaceutical process engineering and economics. *Chimica Oggi-Chemistry Today*, 33:6, 2015.

[61] K. Gilmore, D. Kopetzki, J. W. Lee, Z. Horváth, D. T. McQuade, A. Seidel-Morgenstern, and P. H. Seeberger. Continuous synthesis of artemisinin-derived

medicines. *Chemical Communications*, 50(84):12652–12655, 2014. URL http://dx.doi.org/10.1039/C4CC05098C.

[62] H. Güneş and P. Çalık. Oxygen transfer as a tool for fine-tuning recombinant protein production by *Pichia pastoris* under glyceraldehyde-3-phosphate dehydrogenase promoter. *Bioprocess and Biosystems Engineering*, 39(7):1061–1072, 2016. URL http://doi.org/10.1007/s00449-016-1584-y.

[63] B. Gutmann, D. Cantillo, and C. O. Kappe. Continuous-flow technology–a tool for the safe manufacturing of active pharmaceutical ingredients. *Angewandte Chemie International Edition*, 54(23):6688–6728, 2015. URL http://dx.doi.org/10.1002/anie.201409318.

[64] J. Haber, B. Jiang, T. Maeder, N. Borhani, J. Thome, A. Renken, and L. Kiwi-Minsker. Intensification of highly exothermic fast reaction by multi-injection microstructured reactor. *Chemical Engineering and Processing: Process Intensification*, 84:14–23, 2014. URL http://dx.doi.org/10.1016/j.cep.2014.02.007.

[65] C. Hamel, S. Thomas, K. Schädlich, and A. Seidel-Morgenstern. Theoretical analysis of reactant dosing concepts to perform parallel-series reactions. *Chemical Engineering Science*, 58(19):4483–4492, 2003. URL http://dx.doi.org/10.1016/S0009-2509(03)00308-7.

[66] R. L. Hartman. Managing solids in microreactors for the upstream continuous processing of fine chemicals. *Organic Process Research and Development*, 16(5):870–887, 2012. URL http://pubs.acs.org/doi/10.1021/op200348t.

[67] B. Hentschel, A. Peschel, H. Freund, and K. Sundmacher. Simultaneous design of the optimal reaction and process concept for multiphase systems. *Chemical Engineering Science*, 115:69–87, 2014. URL http://dx.doi.org/10.1016/j.ces.2013.09.046.

[68] V. Hessel. Novel process windows–gate to maximizing process intensification via flow chemistry. *Chemical Engineering & Technology*, 32(11):1655–1681, 2009. URL http://dx.doi.org/10.1002/ceat.200900474.

[69] J. Heyland, J. Fu, L. M. Blank, and A. Schmid. Quantitative physiology of *Pichia pastoris* during glucose-limited high-cell density fed-batch cultivation for recombinant protein production. *Biotechnology and Bioengineering*, 107(2):357–368, 2010. URL http://dx.doi.org/10.1002/bit.22836.

[70] J. Heyland, J. Fu, L. M. Blank, and A. Schmid. Carbon metabolism limits recombinant protein production in *Pichia pastoris*. *Biotechnology and Bioengineering*, 108(8):1942–1953, 2011. URL http://dx.doi.org/10.1002/bit.23114.

[71] F. Hildebrand, S. Kühl, M. Pohl, D. Vasic-Racki, M. Müller, C. Wandrey, and S. Lütz. The production of (R)-2-hydroxy-1-phenyl-propan-1-one derivatives by benzaldehyde lyase from Pseudomonas fluorescens in a continuously operated membrane reactor. *Biotechnology and Bioengineering*, 96(5):835–843, 2007. URL http://doi.wiley.com/10.1002/bit.21189.

[72] D. Hildebrandt and D. Glasser. The attainable region and optimal reactor structures. *Chemical Engineering Science*, 45(8):2161–2168, 1990. URL http://dx.doi.org/10.1016/0009-2509(90)80091-R.

[73] J. L. Hjersted and M. A. Henson. Optimization of fed-batch *Saccharomyces cerevisiae* fermentation using dynamic flux balance models. *Biotechnology Progress*, 22(5):1239–1248, 2006. URL http://dx.doi.org/10.1021/bp060059v.

[74] K. Höffner, S. Harwood, and P. Barton. A reliable simulator for dynamic flux balance analysis. *Biotechnology and Bioengineering*, 110(3):792–802, 2013. URL http://dx.doi.org/10.1002/bit.24748.

[75] HSL. A collection of Fortran codes for large scale scientific computation. 2007. URL http://www.hsl.rl.ac.uk/.

[76] J.-H. Hu, D. White, and H. Johnston. The heat capacity, heat of fusion and heat of vaporization of hydrogen fluoride. *Journal of the American Chemical Society*, 75(5): 1232–1236, 1953. URL http://dx.doi.org/10.1021/ja01101a066.

[77] B. Immel. A Brief History of the GMPs. *Pharmaceutical Technology*, pages 44–52, 2001.

[78] I. A. Isidro, R. M. Portela, J. J. Clemente, A. E. Cunha, and R. Oliveira. Hybrid metabolic flux analysis and recombinant protein prediction in *Pichia pastoris* X-33 cultures expressing a single-chain antibody fragment. *Bioprocess and Biosystems Engineering*, 39(9):1351–1363, 2016. URL http://doi.org/10.1007/s00449-016-1611-z.

[79] K. Jacobs, C. Shoemaker, R. Rudersdorf, S. D. Neill, R. J. Kaufman, A. Mufson, J. Seehra, S. S. Jones, R. Hewick, E. F. Fritsch, et al. Isolation and characterization of genomic and cDNA clones of human erythropoietin. *Nature*, 313(1):806–810, 1985. URL http://dx.doi.org/10.1038/313806a0.

[80] M. Jahic, J. Rotticci-Mulder, M. Martinelle, K. Hult, and S.-O. Enfors. Modeling of growth and energy metabolism of *Pichia pastoris* producing a fusion protein. *Bioprocess and Biosystems Engineering*, 24(6):385–393, 2002. URL https://doi.org/10.1007/s00449-001-0274-5.

[81] C. Jiménez-González, P. Poechlauer, Q. B. Broxterman, B.-S. Yang, D. am Ende, J. Baird, C. Bertsch, R. E. Hannah, P. DellÓrco, H. Noorman, et al. Key green engineering research areas for sustainable manufacturing: A perspective from pharmaceutical and fine chemicals manufacturers. *Organic Process Research & Development*, 15 (4):900–911, 2011. URL http://dx.doi.org/10.1021/op100327d.

[82] M. Jokiel, K. Raetze, N. M. Kaiser, K. U. Künnemann, J.-P. Hollenbeck, J. M. Dreimann, D. Vogt, and K. Sundmacher. Miniplant scale evaluation of a semibatch-continuous tandem reactor system for the hydroformylation of long-chain olefins. *Industrial & Engineering Chemistry Research*, Accepted, 2019.

[83] M. Jokiel, N. M. Kaiser, P. Kováts, M. Mansour, K. Zähringer, K. D. P. Nigam, and K. Sundmacher. Helically coiled segmented flow tubular reactor for the hydroformylation of long-chain olefins in a thermomorphic multiphase system. *Chemical Engineering Journal*, In Press, 2018. URL https://doi.org/10.1016/j.cej.2018.09.221.

[84] H. G. Jolliffe and D. I. Gerogiorgis. Process modelling and simulation for continuous pharmaceutical manufacturing of ibuprofen. *Chemical Engineering Research and Design*, 97:175–191, 2015. URL http://dx.doi.org/10.1016/j.cherd.2014.12.005.

[85] H. G. Jolliffe and D. I. Gerogiorgis. Plantwide design and economic evaluation of two continuous pharmaceutical manufacturing (CPM) cases: ibuprofen and artemisinin. *Computers & Chemical Engineering*, 91:269–288, 2016. URL http://dx.doi.org/10.1016/j.compchemeng.2016.04.005.

[86] H. G. Jolliffe and D. I. Gerogiorgis. Process modelling and simulation for continuous pharmaceutical manufacturing of artemisinin. *Chemical Engineering Research and Design*, 112:310–325, 2016. URL http://dx.doi.org/10.1016/j.cherd.2016.02.017.

[87] J. Joy and A. Kremling. Study of the growth of *Escherichia coli* on mixed substrates using dynamic flux balance analysis. *IFAC Proceedings Volumes*, 43(6):401–406, 2010. URL https://doi.org/10.3182/20100707-3-BE-2012.0059.

[88] C. Jungo, J. Schenk, M. Pasquier, I. W. Marison, and U. von Stockar. A quantitative analysis of the benefits of mixed feeds of sorbitol and methanol for the production of recombinant avidin with *Pichia pastoris*. *Journal of Biotechnology*, 131(1):57–66, 2007. URL http://dx.doi.org/10.1016/j.jbiotec.2007.05.019.

[89] N. M. Kaiser, R. J. Flassig, and K. Sundmacher. Reactor-network synthesis via flux profile analysis. *Chemical Engineering Journal*, 335:1018–1030, 2018. URL http://dx.doi.org/10.1016/j.cej.2017.09.051.

[90] K.-K. K. Kim and R. D. Braatz. Generalised polynomial chaos expansion approaches to approximate stochastic model predictive control. *International Journal of Control*, 86 (8):1324–1337, 2013. URL http://dx.doi.org/10.1080/00207179.2013.801082.

[91] A. A. Kiss, J. Grievink, and M. Rito-Palomares. A systems engineering perspective on process integration in industrial biotechnology. *Journal of Chemical Technology and Biotechnology*, 90(3):349–355, 2015. URL http://doi.wiley.com/10.1002/jctb.4584.

[92] G. Kiss, N. Çelebi-Ölçüm, R. Moretti, D. Baker, and K. N. Houk. Computational enzyme design. *Angewandte Chemie International Edition*, 52(22):5700–5725, 2013. URL http://dx.doi.org/10.1002/anie.201204077.

[93] K. Kobayashi, S. Kuwae, T. Ohya, T. Ohda, M. Ohyama, and K. Tomomitsu. High level secretion of recombinant human serum albumin by fed-batch fermentation of the methylotrophic yeast, *Pichia pastoris*, based on optimal methanol feeding strategy. *Journal of Bioscience and Bioengineering*, 90(3):280–288, 2000. URL https://doi.org/10.1016/S1389-1723(00)80082-1.

[94] N. Kockmann, M. Gottsponer, B. Zimmermann, and D. M. Roberge. Enabling continuous-flow chemistry in microstructured devices for pharmaceutical and fine-chemical production. *Chemistry–A European Journal*, 14(25):7470–7477, 2008. URL http://dx.doi.org/10.1002/chem.200800707.

[95] R. W. Koller, L. A. Ricardez-Sandoval, and L. T. Biegler. Stochastic back-off algorithm for simultaneous design, control, and scheduling of multiproduct systems under uncertainty. *AIChE Journal*, 64(7):2379–2389, 2018. URL http://doi.wiley.com/10.1002/aic.16092.

[96] D. Kumar and H. Budman. Applications of polynomial chaos expansions in optimization and control of bioreactors based on dynamic metabolic flux balance models. *Chemical Engineering Science*, 167:18–28, 2017. URL https://doi.org/10.1016/j.ces.2017.03.035.

[97] J. Kyparisis. On uniqueness of Kuhn-Tucker multipliers in nonlinear programming. *Mathematical Programming*, 32(2):242–246, 1985. URL http://dx.doi.org/10.1007/BF01586095.

[98] R. Lakerveld, B. Benyahia, R. D. Braatz, and P. I. Barton. Model-based design of a plant-wide control strategy for a continuous pharmaceutical plant. *AIChE Journal*, 59 (10):3671–3685, 2013. URL http://dx.doi.org/10.1002/aic.14107.

[99] J. Lalonde. Highly engineered biocatalysts for efficient small molecule pharmaceutical synthesis. *Current Opinion in Biotechnology*, 42:152–158, 2016. URL http://dx.doi.org/10.1016/j.copbio.2016.04.023.

[100] J. W. Lee, Z. Horvath, A. G. O'Brien, P. H. Seeberger, and A. Seidel-Morgenstern. Design and optimization of coupling a continuously operated reactor with simulated moving bed chromatography. *Chemical Engineering Journal*, 251:355–370, 2014. URL http://doi.wiley.com/10.1016/j.cej.2014.04.043.

[101] U. N. Lerner. *Hybrid Bayesian networks for reasoning about complex systems*. PhD thesis, Stanford University, Stanford, CA, 2002.

[102] D. Li, Q. Wang, J. Wang, and Y. Yao. Mitigation of curse of dimensionality in dynamic programming. *IFAC Proceedings Volumes*, 41(2):7778–7783, 2008. URL https://doi.org/10.3182/20080706-5-KR-1001.01315.

[103] F. Llaneras, M. Tortajada, D. Ramón, and J. Picó. Dynamic metabolic flux analysis for online estimation of recombinant protein productivity in *Pichia pastoris* cultures. *IFAC Proceedings Volumes*, 45(2):629–634, 2012. URL http://dx.doi.org/10.3182/20120215-3-AT-3016.00112.

[104] F. Logist, I. Smets, and J. Van Impe. Derivation of generic optimal reference temperature profiles for steady-state exothermic jacketed tubular reactors. *Journal of Process*

Control, 18(1):92–104, 2008. URL https://doi.org/10.1016/j.jprocont.2007.05.001.

[105] J. C. Love, K. R. Love, and P. W. Barone. Enabling global access to high-quality biopharmaceuticals. *Current Opinion in Chemical Engineering*, 2(4):383–390, 2013. URL http://dx.doi.org/10.1016/j.coche.2013.09.002.

[106] A. E. Lu, J. A. Paulson, N. J. Mozdzierz, A. Stockdale, A. N. F. Versypt, K. R. Love, J. C. Love, and R. D. Braatz. Control systems technology in the advanced manufacturing of biologic drugs. In *Control Applications (CCA), 2015 IEEE Conference on*, pages 1505–1515. IEEE, 2015. URL http://dx.doi.org/10.1109/CCA.2015.7320824.

[107] Y. Lu, A. G. Dixon, W. R. Moser, and Y. H. Ma. Analysis and optimization of cross-flow reactors with staged feed policies–isothermal operation with parallel-series, irreversible reaction systems. *Chemical Engineering Science*, 52(8):1349–1363, 1997. URL http://dx.doi.org/10.1016/S0009-2509(96)00491-5.

[108] R. Mahadevan, J. S. Edwards, and F. J. Doyle. Dynamic flux balance analysis of diauxic growth in *Escherichia coli*. *Biophysical Journal*, 83(3):1331–1340, 2002. URL http://dx.doi.org/10.1016/S0006-3495(02)73903-9.

[109] F. Marpani, Z. Sárossy, M. Pinelo, and A. S. Meyer. Kinetics based reaction optimization of enzyme catalyzed reduction of formaldehyde to methanol with synchronous cofactor regeneration. *Biotechnology and Bioengineering*, 114(12):2762–2770, 2017. URL http://doi.wiley.com/10.1002/bit.26405.

[110] S. Mascia, P. L. Heider, H. Zhang, R. Lakerveld, B. Benyahia, P. I. Barton, R. D. Braatz, C. L. Cooney, J. Evans, T. F. Jamison, et al. End-to-end continuous manufacturing of pharmaceuticals: Integrated synthesis, purification, and final dosage formation. *Angewandte Chemie International Edition*, 52(47):12359–12363, 2013. URL http://dx.doi.org/10.1002/anie.201305429.

[111] A. L. Meadows, R. Karnik, H. Lam, S. Forestell, and B. Snedecor. Application of dynamic flux balance analysis to an industrial *Escherichia coli* fermentation. *Metabolic Engineering*, 12(2):150–160, 2010. URL http://dx.doi.org/10.1016/j.ymben.2009.07.006.

[112] H. Menard, R. Beaudoin, and K. Loczy. Measurements of ro (h) and ro (f) in alcohol hydrogen fluoride mixtures. *Journal of Chemical and Engineering Data*, 29(2):120–121, 1984. URL http://dx.doi.org/10.1021/je00036a004.

[113] A. Mesbah, S. Streif, R. Findeisen, and R. D. Braatz. Stochastic nonlinear model predictive control with probabilistic constraints. *2014 American Control Conference*, pages 2413–2419, 2014. URL http://dx.doi.org/10.1109/ACC.2014.6858851.

[114] R. E. Mesmer and B. F. Hitch. Base strength of amines at high temperatures. Ionization of cyclohexylamine and morpholine. *Journal of Solution Chemistry*, 6(4):251–261, 1977. URL http://dx.doi.org/10.1007/BF00645456.

[115] Y. Morales, M. Tortajada, J. Picó, J. Vehí, and F. Llaneras. Validation of an FBA model for *Pichia pastoris* in chemostat cultures. *BMC Systems Biology*, 8:142, 2014. URL http://dx.doi.org/10.1186/s12918-014-0142-y.

[116] R. Morales-Rodriguez, A. S. Meyer, K. V. Gernaey, and G. Sin. A framework for model-based optimization of bioprocesses under uncertainty: Lignocellulosic ethanol production case. *Computers & Chemical Engineering*, 42:115–129, 2012. URL http://dx.doi.org/10.1016/j.compchemeng.2011.12.004.

[117] N. J. Mozdzierz, K. R. Love, K. S. Lee, H. L. Lee, K. A. Shah, R. J. Ram, and J. C. Love. A perfusion-capable microfluidic bioreactor for assessing microbial heterologous protein production. *Lab on a Chip*, 15(14):2918–2922, 2015. URL http://dx.doi.org/10.1039/C5LC00443H.

[118] M. Müller, G. A. Sprenger, and M. Pohl. C–C bond formation using ThDP-dependent lyases. *Current Opinion in Chemical Biology*, 17(2):261–270, 2013. URL https://doi.org/10.1016/j.cbpa.2013.02.017.

[119] D. F. M. Muñoz, N. A. A. Enciso, H. C. Ruiz, and L. A. B. Avellaneda. A simple structured model for recombinant IDShr protein production in *Pichia pastoris*. *Biotechnology Letters*, 30(10):1727–1734, 2008. URL http://dx.doi.org/10.1007/s10529-008-9750-1.

[120] K. D. Nagy, B. Shen, T. F. Jamison, and K. F. Jensen. Mixing and dispersion in small–scale flow systems. *Organic Process Research & Development*, 16(5):976–981, 2012. URL http://dx.doi.org/10.1021/op200349f.

[121] H. Niu, M. Daukandt, C. Rodriguez, P. Fickers, and P. Bogaerts. Dynamic modeling of methylotrophic *Pichia pastoris* culture with exhaust gas analysis: From cellular metabolism to process simulation. *Chemical Engineering Science*, 87:381–392, 2013. URL http://dx.doi.org/10.1016/j.ces.2012.11.006.

[122] J. Nocon, M. G. Steiger, M. Pfeffer, S. B. Sohn, T. Y. Kim, M. Maurer, H. Rußmayer, S. Pflügl, M. Ask, C. Haberhauer-Troyer, et al. Model based engineering of *Pichia pastoris* central metabolism enhances recombinant protein production. *Metabolic Engineering*, 24:129–138, 2014. URL http://dx.doi.org/10.1016/j.ymben.2014.05.011.

[123] A. G. O'Brien, Z. Horváth, F. Lévesque, J. W. Lee, A. Seidel-Morgenstern, and P. H. Seeberger. Continuous synthesis and purification by direct coupling of a flow reactor with simulated moving-bed chromatography. *Angewandte Chemie International Edition*, 51(28):7028–7030, 2012. URL http://doi.wiley.com/10.1002/anie.201202795.

[124] R. Ohs, J. Wendlandt, and A. C. Spiess. How graphical analysis helps interpreting optimal experimental designs for nonlinear enzyme kinetic models. *AIChE Journal*, 63(11):4870–4880, 2017. URL http://dx.doi.org/10.1002/aic.15814.

[125] R. Ohs, K. Fischer, M. Schoepping, and A. C. Spiess. Development of a mechanistic model for a branched enzyme-catalyzed carboligation. Submitted, 2018.

[126] R. Ohs, M. Leipnitz, M. Schöpping, and A. C. Spiess. Simultaneous identification of reaction and inactivation kinetics of an enzyme-catalyzed carboligation. *Biotechnology Progress*, pages 1–34, 2018. URL http://doi.wiley.com/10.1002/btpr.2656.

[127] J. D. Orth, I. Thiele, and B. Ø. Palsson. What is flux balance analysis? *Nature Biotechnology*, 28(3):245–248. URL http://dx.doi.org/10.1038/nbt.1614.

[128] L. Özkan, T. Backx, T. Van Gerven, and A. Stankiewicz. Towards Perfect Reactors: Gaining full control of chemical transformations at molecular level. *Chemical Engineering and Processing: Process Intensification*, 51:109–116, 2012. URL http://dx.doi.org/10.1016/j.cep.2011.09.013.

[129] S. Park and W. Fred Ramirez. Optimal production of secreted protein in fed-batch reactors. *AIChE Journal*, 34(9):1550–1558, 1988. URL https://doi.org/10.1002/aic.690340917.

[130] J. A. Paulson and A. Mesbah. An efficient method for stochastic optimal control with joint chance constraints for nonlinear systems. *International Journal of Robust and Nonlinear Control*, (October):1–21, 2017. URL http://doi.wiley.com/10.1002/rnc.3999.

[131] A. Peschel. *Model-based Design of Optimal Chemical Reactors*. Shaker Verlag, Aachen, 2012.

[132] A. Peschel, H. Freund, and K. Sundmacher. Methodology for the design of optimal chemical reactors based on the concept of elementary process functions. *Industrial & Engineering Chemistry Research*, 49(21):10535–10548, 2010. URL http://dx.doi.org/10.1021/ie100476q.

[133] A. Peschel, F. Karst, H. Freund, and K. Sundmacher. Analysis and optimal design of an ethylene oxide reactor. *Chemical Engineering Science*, 66(24):6453–6469, 2011. URL http://dx.doi.org/10.1016/j.ces.2011.08.054.

[134] A. Peschel, B. Hentschel, H. Freund, and K. Sundmacher. Design of optimal multiphase reactors exemplified on the hydroformylation of long chain alkenes. *Chemical Engineering Journal*, 188:126–141, 2012. URL http://dx.doi.org/10.1016/j.cej.2012.01.123.

[135] T. Ploch. Model-based optimization of an enzyme-catalyzed reaction network. Master's thesis, Rheinisch-Westfälische Technische Hochschule Aachen, Aachen, Germany, 2014.

[136] P. Plouffe, A. Macchi, and D. M. Roberge. From batch to continuous chemical synthesis– a toolbox approach. *Organic Process Research & Development*, 18(11):1286–1294, 2014. URL http://dx.doi.org/10.1021/op5001918.

[137] D. J. Pollard and J. M. Woodley. Biocatalysis for pharmaceutical intermediates: the future is now. *Trends in Biotechnology*, 25(2):66–73, 2007. URL https://doi.org/10.1016/j.tibtech.2006.12.005.

[138] L. S. Pontryagin, V. G. Boltyanskii, R. F. Gamkrelidze, and E. F. Mishechenko. *Mathematical Theory of Optimal Processes*. Wiley, New York, 1962.

[139] G. Potvin, A. Ahmad, and Z. Zhang. Bioprocess engineering aspects of heterologous protein production in *Pichia pastoris*: a review. *Biochemical Engineering Journal*, 64: 91–105, 2012. URL http://dx.doi.org/10.1016/j.bej.2010.07.017.

[140] J. Price, B. Hofmann, V. T. L. Silva, M. Nordblad, J. M. Woodley, and J. K. Huusom. Mechanistic modeling of biodiesel production using a liquid lipase formulation. *Biotechnology Progress*, 30(6):1277–1290, 2014. URL http://doi.wiley.com/10.1002/btpr.1985.

[141] J. Puschke, A. Zubov, J. Kosek, and A. Mitsos. Multi-model approach based on parametric sensitivities – A heuristic approximation for dynamic optimization of semi-batch processes with parametric uncertainties. *Computers & Chemical Engineering*, 98: 161–179, 2017. URL http://dx.doi.org/10.1016/j.compchemeng.2016.12.004.

[142] A. U. Raghunathan, J. R. Pérez-Correa, and L. T. Bieger. Data reconciliation and parameter estimation in flux-balance analysis. *Biotechnology and Bioengineering*, 84(6): 700–709, 2003. URL http://dx.doi.org/10.1002/bit.10823.

[143] D. Ralph and S. J. Wright. Some properties of regularization and penalization schemes for MPECs. *Optimization Methods and Software*, 19(5):527–556, 2004. URL http://dx.doi.org/10.1080/10556780410001709439.

[144] J. Rantanen and J. Khinast. The future of pharmaceutical manufacturing sciences. *Journal of Pharmaceutical Sciences*, 104(11):3612–3638, 2015. URL http://dx.doi.org/10.1002/jps.24594.

[145] B. J. Reizman and K. F. Jensen. An automated continuous-flow platform for the estimation of multistep reaction kinetics. *Organic Process Research & Development*, 16 (11):1770–1782, 2012. URL http://dx.doi.org/10.1021/op3001838.

[146] H. T. Ren, J. Q. Yuan, and K. H. Bellgardt. Macrokinetic model for methylotrophic *Pichia pastoris* based on stoichiometric balance. *Journal of Biotechnology*, 106(1):53–68, 2003. URL http://dx.doi.org/10.1016/j.jbiotec.2003.08.003.

[147] D. N. Rihani and L. K. Doraiswamy. Estimation of heat capacity of organic compounds from group contributions. *Industrial & Engineering Chemistry Fundamentals*, 4 (1):17–21, 1965. URL http://dx.doi.org/10.1021/i160013a003.

[148] R. H. Ringborg and J. M. Woodley. The application of reaction engineering to biocatalysis. *React. Chem. Eng.*, 1(1):10–22, 2016. URL http://xlink.rsc.org/?DOI=C5RE00045A.

[149] D. Roberge. Lonza–hazardous flow chemistry for streamlined large scale synthesis. *Green Processing and Synthesis*, 1(1):129–130, 2012. URL http://dx.doi.org/10.1515/greenps-2011-0504.

[150] D. M. Roberge. The complexity of technology implementation: flow versus batch processing. *Chimica Oggi-Chemistry Today*, 30:5, 2012.

[151] D. M. Roberge. What is flow chemistry? *Chimica Oggi-Chemistry Today*, 33:4, 2015.

[152] D. M. Roberge, N. Bieler, M. Mathier, M. Eyholzer, B. Zimmermann, P. Barthe, C. Guermeur, O. Lobet, M. Moreno, and P. Woehl. Development of an industrial multi-injection microreactor for fast and exothermic reactions–part II. *Chemical Engineering & Technology*, 31(8):1155–1161, 2008. URL http://dx.doi.org/10.1002/ceat.200800131.

[153] D. M. Roberge, B. Zimmermann, F. Rainone, M. Gottsponer, M. Eyholzer, and N. Kockmann. Microreactor technology and continuous processes in the fine chemical and pharmaceutical industry: is the revolution underway? *Organic Process Research & Development*, 12(5):905–910, 2008. URL http://dx.doi.org/10.1021/op8001273.

[154] P. A. Romero, A. Krause, and F. H. Arnold. Navigating the protein fitness landscape with Gaussian processes. *Proceedings of the National Academy of Sciences*, 110(3):E193–E201, 2013. URL http://www.pnas.org/cgi/doi/10.1073/pnas.1215251110.

[155] S. Sager. Reformulations and algorithms for the optimization of switching decisions in nonlinear optimal control. *Journal of Process Control*, 19(8):1238–1247, 2009. URL http://doi.org/10.1016/j.jprocont.2009.03.008.

[156] F. Saitua, P. Torres, J. R. Pérez-Correa, and E. Agosin. Dynamic genome-scale metabolic modeling of the yeast *Pichia pastoris*. *BMC Systems Biology*, 11:27, 2017. URL http://dx.doi.org/10.1186/s12918-017-0408-2.

[157] B. J. Sánchez, J. R. Pérez-Correa, and E. Agosin. Construction of robust dynamic genome-scale metabolic model structures of *Saccharomyces cerevisiae* through iterative re-parameterization. *Metabolic Engineering*, 25:159–173, 2014. URL http://dx.doi.org/10.1016/j.ymben.2014.07.004.

[158] S. D. Schaber, D. I. Gerogiorgis, R. Ramachandran, J. M. B. Evans, P. I. Barton, and B. L. Trout. Economic analysis of integrated continuous and batch pharmaceutical manufacturing: a case study. *Industrial & Engineering Chemistry Research*, 50(17): 10083–10092, 2011. URL http://dx.doi.org/10.1021/ie2006752.

[159] R. Schenkendorf. A general framework for uncertainty propagation based on point estimate methods. *Second European Conference of the Prognostics and Health Management Society, PHME14*, 2014.

[160] R. Schenkendorf. Supporting the shift towards continuous pharmaceutical manufacturing by condition monitoring. *Conference on Control and Fault-Tolerant Systems, SysTol*, 2016-November:593–598, 2016. URL http://dx.doi.org/10.1109/SYSTOL.2016.7739813.

[161] R. Schenkendorf, X. Xie, M. Rehbein, S. Scholl, and U. Krewer. The impact of global sensitivities and design measures in model-based optimal experimental design. *Processes*, 6(4):27, 2018. URL http://dx.doi.org/10.3390/pr6040027.

[162] M. Schiestl, T. Stangler, C. Torella, T. Čepeljnik, H. Toll, and R. Grau. Acceptable changes in quality attributes of glycosylated biopharmaceuticals. *Nature Biotechnology*, 29(4):310–312, 2011. URL http://dx.doi.org/10.1038/nbt.1839.

[163] R. Schuetz, L. Kuepfer, and U. Sauer. Systematic evaluation of objective functions for predicting intracellular fluxes in *Escherichia coli*. *Molecular Systems Biology*, 3:119, 2007. URL http://dx.doi.org/10.1038/msb4100162.

[164] D. Segre, D. Vitkup, and G. M. Church. Analysis of optimality in natural and perturbed metabolic networks. *Proceedings of the National Academy of Sciences*, 99(23): 15112–15117, 2002. URL http://dx.doi.org/10.1073/pnas.232349399.

[165] J. Shi, L. T. Biegler, I. Hamdan, and J. Wassick. Optimization of grade transitions in polyethylene solution polymerization process under uncertainty. *Computers & Chemical Engineering*, 95:260–279, 2016. URL http://dx.doi.org/10.1016/j.compchemeng.2016.08.002.

[166] C. A. Shukla, A. A. Kulkarni, and V. V. Ranade. Selectivity engineering of the diazotization reaction in a continuous flow reactor. *Reaction Chemistry & Engineering*, 2016. URL http://dx.doi.org/10.1039/C5RE00056D.

[167] L. L. Simon, H. Pataki, G. Marosi, F. Meemken, K. Hungerbühler, A. Baiker, S. Tummala, B. Glennon, M. Kuentz, G. Steele, H. J. Kramer, J. W. Rydzak, Z. Chen, J. Morris, F. Kjell, R. Singh, R. Gani, K. V. Gernaey, M. Louhi-Kultanen, J. Oreilly, N. Sandler, O. Antikainen, J. Yliruusi, P. Frohberg, J. Ulrich, R. D. Braatz, T. Leyssens, M. Von Stosch, R. Oliveira, R. B. Tan, H. Wu, M. Khan, D. Ogrady, A. Pandey, R. Westra, E. Delle-Case, D. Pape, D. Angelosante, Y. Maret, O. Steiger, M. Lenner, K. Abbou-Oucherif, Z. K. Nagy, J. D. Litster, V. K. Kamaraju, and M. S. Chiu. Assessment of recent process analytical technology (PAT) trends: A multiauthor review. *Organic Process Research and Development*, 19(1):3–62, 2015. URL http://dx.doi.org/10.1021/op500261y.

[168] G. Sin, K. V. Gernaey, and A. E. Lantz. Good modelling practice (GMoP) for PAT applications: Propagation of input uncertainty and sensitivity analysis. *Biotechnology Progress*, 25:1043–1053, 2009. URL http://dx.doi.org/10.1021/bp.166.

[169] I. Y. Smets, D. Dochain, and J. F. Van Impe. Optimal temperature control of a steady-state exothermic plug-flow reactor. *AIChE Journal*, 48(2):279–286, 2002. URL https://onlinelibrary.wiley.com/doi/abs/10.1002/aic.690480212.

[170] D. R. Snead and T. F. Jamison. End-to-end continuous flow synthesis and purification of diphenhydramine hydrochloride featuring atom economy, in-line separation, and flow of molten ammonium salts. *Chemical Science*, 4(7):2822–2827, 2013. URL http://dx.doi.org/10.1039/C3SC50859E.

[171] A. Solà, P. Jouhten, H. Maaheimo, F. Sanchez-Ferrando, T. Szyperski, and P. Ferrer. Metabolic flux profiling of *Pichia pastoris* grown on glycerol/methanol mixtures in chemostat cultures at low and high dilution rates. *Microbiology*, 153(1):281–290, 2007. URL https://doi.org/10.1099/mic.0.29263-0.

[172] K. Sreekrishna, R. G. Brankamp, K. E. Kropp, D. T. Blankenship, J.-T. Tsay, P. L. Smith, J. D. Wierschke, A. Subramaniam, and L. A. Birkenberger. Strategies for optimal synthesis and secretion of heterologous proteins in the methylotrophic yeast *Pichia pastoris*. *Gene*, 190(1):55–62, 1997. URL http://dx.doi.org/10.1016/S0378-1119(96)00672-5.

[173] B. Srinivasan, D. Bonvin, E. Visser, and S. Palanki. Dynamic optimization of batch processes: II. Role of measurements in handling uncertainty. *Computers & Chemical Engineering*, 27(1):27–44, 2003. URL http://dx.doi.org/10.1016/S0098-1354(02)00117-5.

[174] P. C. St. John, M. F. Crowley, and Y. J. Bomble. Efficient estimation of the maximum metabolic productivity of batch systems. *Biotechnology for Biofuels*, 10:28, 2017. URL https://doi.org/10.1186/s13068-017-0709-0.

[175] A. I. Stankiewicz, J. A. Moulijn, et al. Process intensification: transforming chemical engineering. *Chemical Engineering Progress*, 96(1):22–34, 2000.

[176] T. Stillger, M. Pohl, C. Wandrey, and A. Liese. Reaction engineering of benzaldehyde lyase from *Pseudomonas fluorescens* catalyzing enantioselective C-C bond formation. *Organic Process Research & Development*, 10(15):1172–1177, 2006. URL http://pubs.acs.org/doi/abs/10.1021/op0601316.

[177] P. Stonestreet and A. Harvey. A mixing-based design methodology for continuous oscillatory flow reactors. *Chemical Engineering Research and Design*, 80(1):31–44, 2002. URL http://dx.doi.org/10.1205/026387602753393204.

[178] S. Streif, K. K. K. Kim, P. Rumschinski, M. Kishida, D. E. Shen, R. Findeisen, and R. D. Braatz. Robustness analysis, prediction, and estimation for uncertain biochemical networks: An overview. *Journal of Process Control*, 42:14–34, 2016. URL http://dx.doi.org/10.1016/j.jprocont.2016.03.004.

[179] J. P. Swann. The 1941 sulfathiazole disaster and the birth of good manufacturing practices. *Pharmacy in History*, 41(1):16–25, 1999.

[180] D. Telen, M. Vallerio, L. Cabianca, B. Houska, J. Van Impe, and F. Logist. Approximate robust optimization of nonlinear systems under parametric uncertainty and process noise. *Journal of Process Control*, 33:140–154, 2015. URL http://dx.doi.org/10.1016/j.jprocont.2015.06.011.

[181] I. Thiele and B. Ø. Palsson. A protocol for generating a high-quality genome-scale metabolic reconstruction. *Nature Protocols*, 5(1):93–121, 2010. URL http://dx.doi.org/10.1038/nprot.2009.203.

[182] G. M. Troup and C. Georgakis. Process systems engineering tools in the pharmaceutical industry. *Computers and Chemical Engineering*, 51:157–171, 2013. URL http://dx.doi.org/10.1016/j.compchemeng.2012.06.014.

[183] E. Tziampazis and A. Sambanis. Modeling of cell culture processes. *Cytotechnology*, 14(3):191–204, 1994. URL http://dx.doi.org/10.1007/BF00749616.

[184] F. E. Valera, M. Quaranta, A. Moran, J. Blacker, A. Armstrong, J. T. Cabral, and D. G. Blackmond. The flow's the thing...or is it? assessing the merits of homogeneous reactions in flask and flow. *Angewandte Chemie International Edition*, 49(14):2478–2485, 2010. URL http://doi.wiley.com/10.1002/anie.200906095.

[185] V. S. Vassiliadis, R. W. Sargent, and C. C. Pantelides. Solution of a class of multistage dynamic optimization problems. 1. problems without path constraints. *Industrial & Engineering Chemistry Research*, 33(9):2111–2122, 1994. URL http://doi.org/10.1021/ie00033a014.

[186] V. S. Vassiliadis, R. W. H. Sargent, and C. C. Pantelides. Solution of a class of multistage dynamic optimization problems. 2. problems with path constraints. *Industrial & Engineering Chemistry Research*, 33:2123–2123, 1994. URL http://doi.org/10.1021/ie00033a015.

[187] D. Vercammen, F. Logist, and J. Van Impe. Dynamic estimation of specific fluxes in metabolic networks using non-linear dynamic optimization. *BMC Systems Biology*, 8: 132, 2014. URL https://doi.org/10.1186/s12918-014-0132-0.

[188] D. Vercammen, D. Telen, P. Nimmegeers, A. Janssens, S. Akkermans, E. N. Fernandez, F. Logist, and J. Van Impe. Application of a dynamic metabolic flux algorithm during a temperature-induced lag phase. *Food and Bioproducts Processing*, 102:1–19, 2017. URL http://doi.org/10.1016/j.fbp.2016.10.003.

[189] E. Visser, B. Srinivasan, S. Palanki, and D. Bonvin. A feedback-based implementation scheme for batch process optimization. *Journal of Process Control*, 10:399–410, 2000. URL http://dx.doi.org/10.1016/S0959-1524(00)00015-9.

[190] G. Wachsmuth. On LICQ and the uniqueness of Lagrange multipliers. *Operations Research Letters*, 41(1):78–80, 2013. URL http://dx.doi.org/10.1016/j.orl.2012.11.009.

[191] A. Wächter and L. T. Biegler. On the implementation of an interior-point filter line-search algorithm for large-scale nonlinear programming. *Mathematical Programming*, 106(1):25–57, 2006. URL https://doi.org/10.1007/s10107-004-0559-y.

[192] S. Waldherr. State estimation in constraint based models of metabolic-genetic networks. In *American Control Conference (ACC), 2016*, pages 6683–6688. IEEE, 2016. URL http://doi.org/10.1109/ACC.2016.7526723.

[193] G. Walsh. Biopharmaceutical benchmarks 2014. *Nature Biotechnology*, 32(10):992–1000, 2014. URL http://dx.doi.org/http://dx.doi.org/10.1038/nbt.3040.

[194] S. Wegerhoff and S. Engell. Control of the production of *Saccharomyces cerevisiae* on the basis of a reduced metabolic model. *IFAC-PapersOnLine*, 49(26):201–206, 2016. URL https://doi.org/10.1016/j.ifacol.2016.12.126.

[195] E. Wells and A. S. Robinson. Cellular engineering for therapeutic protein production: product quality, host modification, and process improvement. *Biotechnology Journal*, 12(1):1860–7314, 2017. URL http://dx.doi.org/10.1002/biot.201600105.

[196] T. Westermann and L. Mleczko. Heat management in microreactors for fast exothermic organic syntheses–first design principles. *Organic Process Research & Development*, 20(2):487–494, 2016. URL http://dx.doi.org/10.1021/acs.oprd.5b00205.

[197] C. Wiles and P. Watts. Improving chemical synthesis using flow reactors. *Expert Opinion on Drug Discovery*, 2(11):1487–1503, 2007. URL http://dx.doi.org/10.1517/17460441.2.11.1487.

[198] P. M. Witt, S. Somasi, I. Khan, D. W. Blaylock, J. A. Newby, and S. V. Ley. Modeling mesoscale reactors for the production of fine chemicals. *Chemical Engineering Journal*, 278:353–362, 2015. URL http://dx.doi.org/10.1016/j.cej.2014.12.030.

[199] J. M. Woodley. New opportunities for biocatalysis: making pharmaceutical processes greener. *Trends in Biotechnology*, 26(6):321–327, 2008. URL https://doi.org/10.1016/j.tibtech.2008.03.004.

[200] J. M. Woodley. Bioprocess intensification for the effective production of chemical products. *Computers & Chemical Engineering*, 105:297–307, 2017. URL http://dx.doi.org/10.1016/j.compchemeng.2017.01.015.

[201] J. M. Woodley. Integrating protein engineering with process design for biocatalysis. *Philosophical Transactions of the Royal Society A: Mathematical, Physical and Engineering Sciences*, 376(2110):20170062, 2018. URL https://doi.org/10.1098/rsta.2017.0062.

[202] J. Xie, Q. Zhou, P. Du, R. Gan, and Q. Ye. Use of different carbon sources in cultivation of recombinant *Pichia pastoris* for angiostatin production. *Enzyme and Microbial Technology*, 36(2):210–216, 2005. URL http://dx.doi.org/10.1016/j.enzmictec.2004.06.010.

[203] M. Xie and H. Freund. Fast synthesis of optimal chemical reactor networks based on a universal system representation. *Chemical Engineering and Processing: Process Intensification*, 123:280–290, 2018. URL https://doi.org/10.1016/j.cep.2017.11.011.

[204] X. Xie, U. Krewer, and R. Schenkendorf. Robust optimization of dynamical systems with correlated random variables using the point estimate method. *IFAC-PapersOnLine*, 51(2):427–432, 2018. URL https://doi.org/10.1016/j.ifacol.2018.03.073.

[205] L. Yang, R. Mahadevan, and W. R. Cluett. A bilevel optimization algorithm to identify enzymatic capacity constraints in metabolic networks. *Computers & Chemical Engineering*, 32(9):2072–2085, 2008. URL http://doi.org/10.1016/j.compchemeng.2007.10.015.

[206] M. Zavrel, T. Schmidt, C. Michalik, M. Ansorge-Schumacher, W. Marquardt, J. Büchs, and A. C. Spiess. Mechanistic kinetic model for symmetric carboligations using benzaldehyde lyase. *Biotechnology and Bioengineering*, 101(1):27–38, 2008. URL http://doi.wiley.com/10.1002/bit.21867.

[207] W. Zhang, M. A. Bevins, B. A. Plantz, L. A. Smith, and M. M. Meagher. Modeling *Pichia pastoris* growth on methanol and optimizing the production of a recombinant protein, the heavy-chain fragment C of botulinum neurotoxin, serotype A. *Biotechnology and Bioengineering*, 70(1):1–8, 2000. URL http://dx.doi.org/10.1002/1097-0290(20001005)70:1<1::AID-BIT1>3.0.CO;2-Y.

[208] X. Zhao, S. Noack, W. Wiechert, and E. von Lieres. Dynamic flux balance analysis with nonlinear objective function. *Journal of Mathematical Biology*, 75(6-7):1487–1515, 2017. URL https://doi.org/10.1007/s00285-017-1127-4.

INDEX